Recent Advances in Laparoscopic Surgery

Edited by Francisco M. Sánchez Margallo and Juan A. Sánchez-Margallo

Published in London, United Kingdom

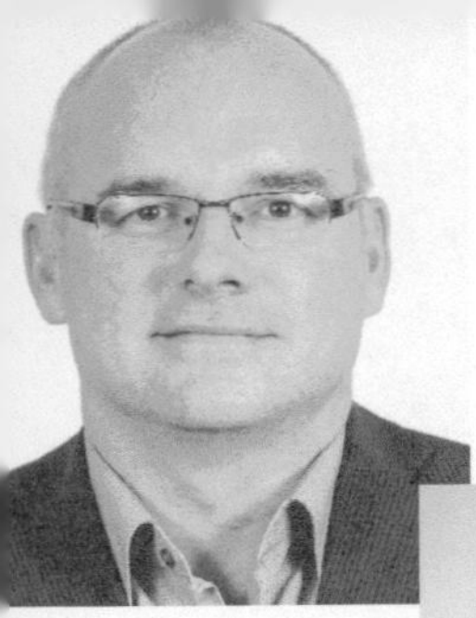
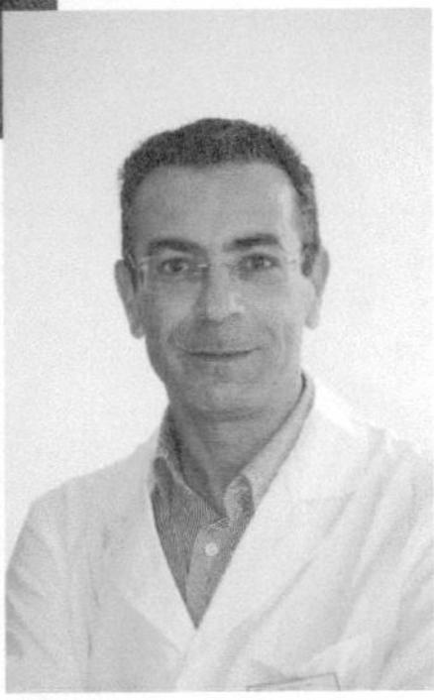
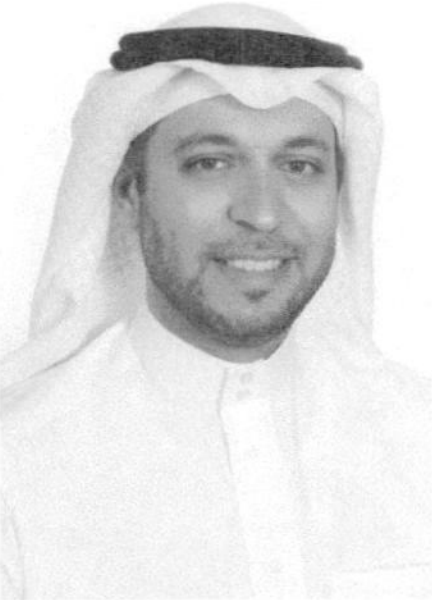
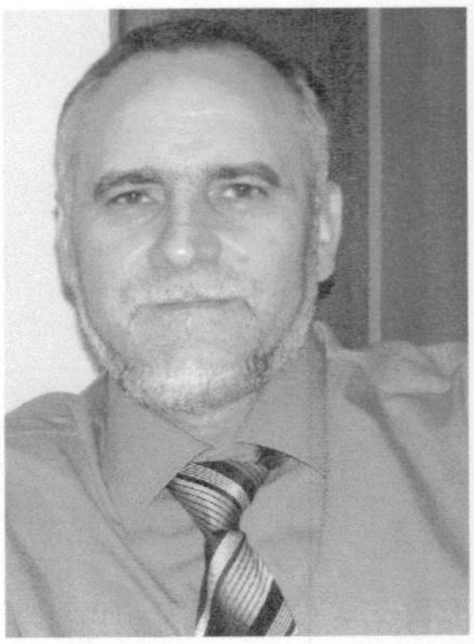
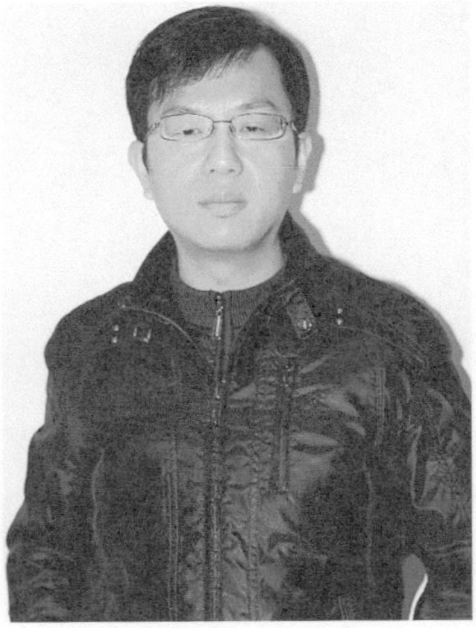
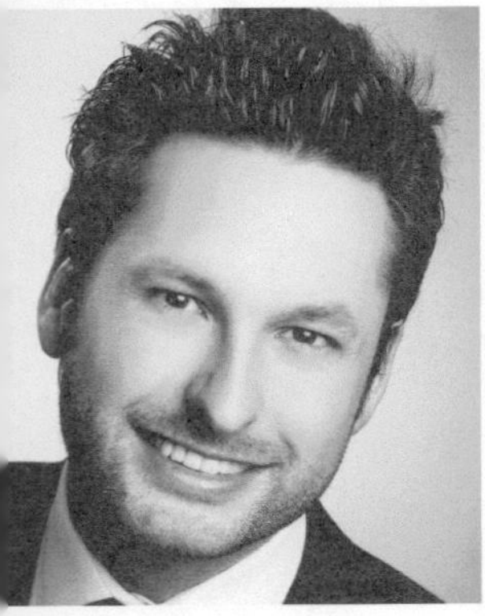
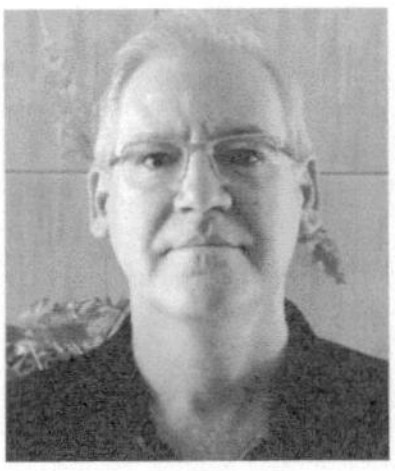

IntechOpen

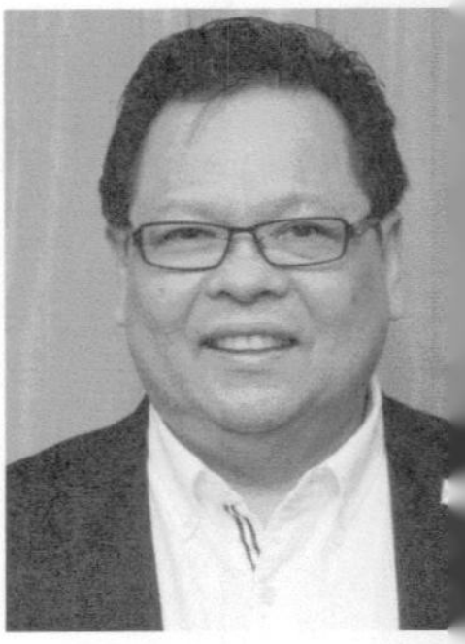
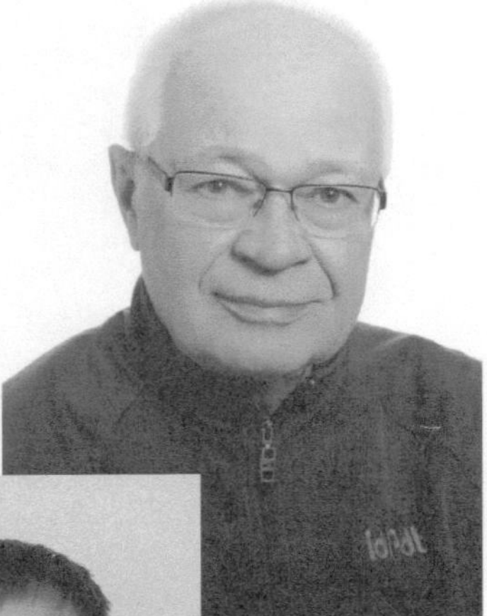
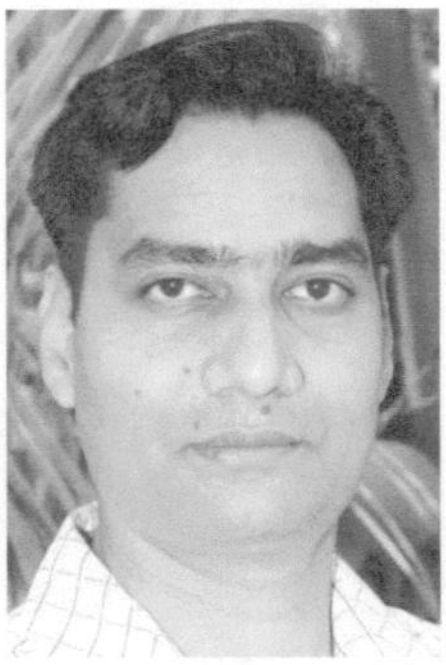
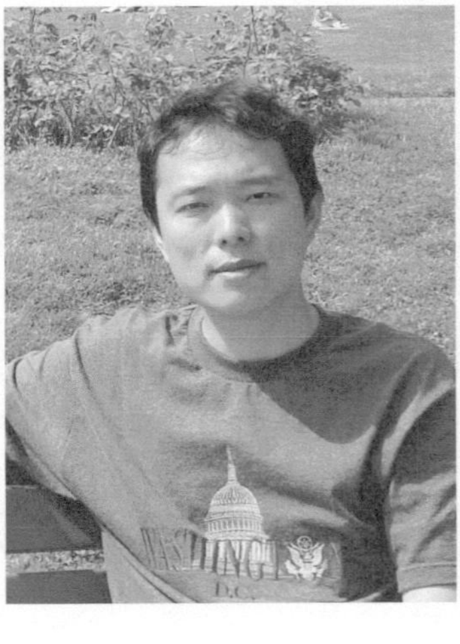
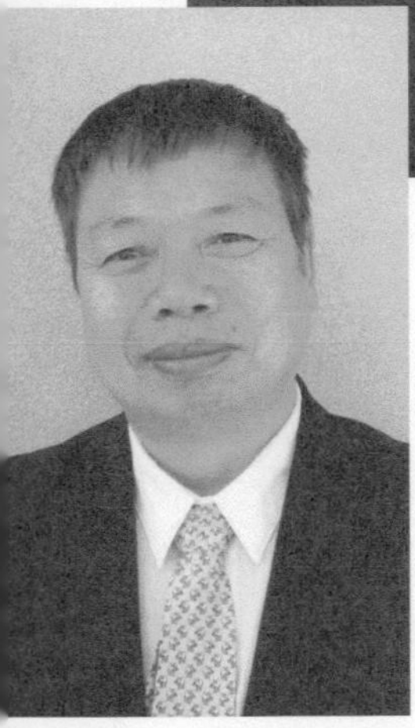
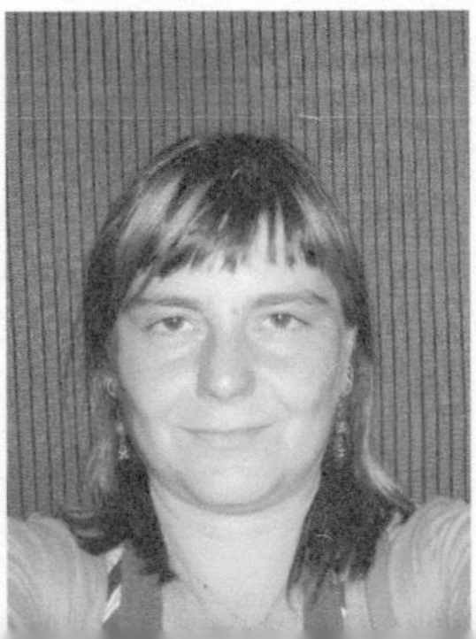

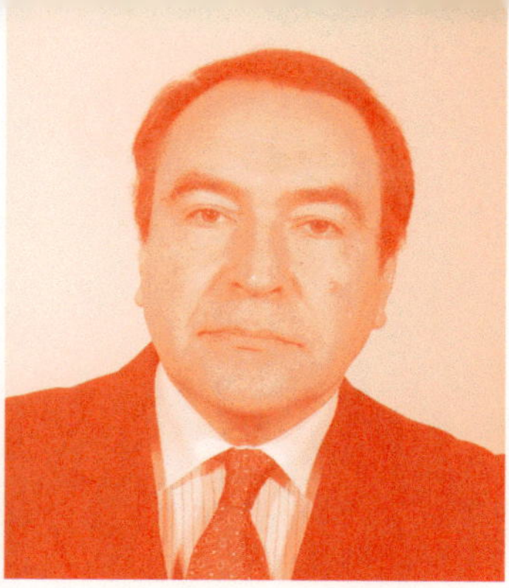
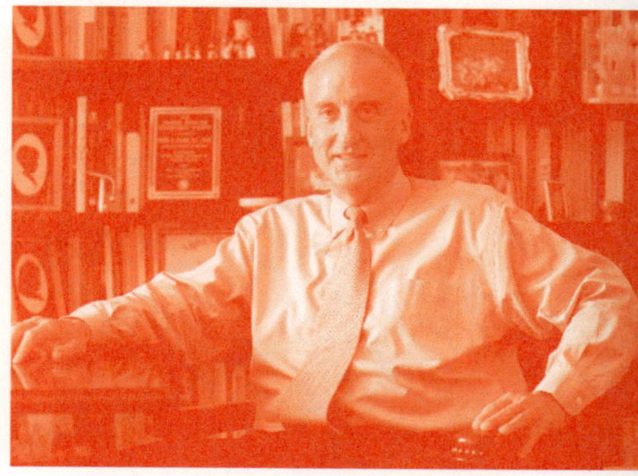
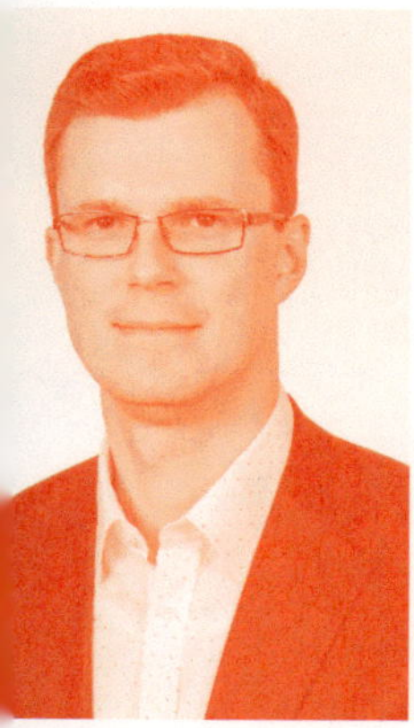
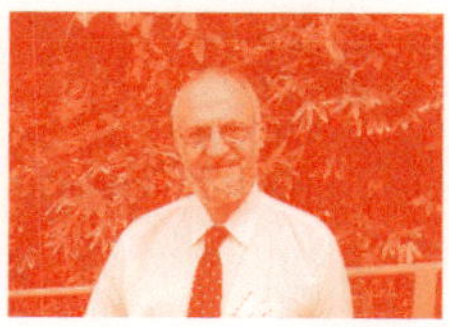
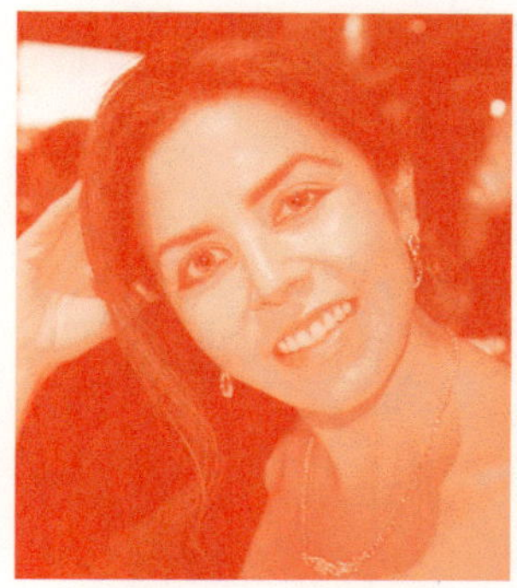

Supporting open minds since 2005

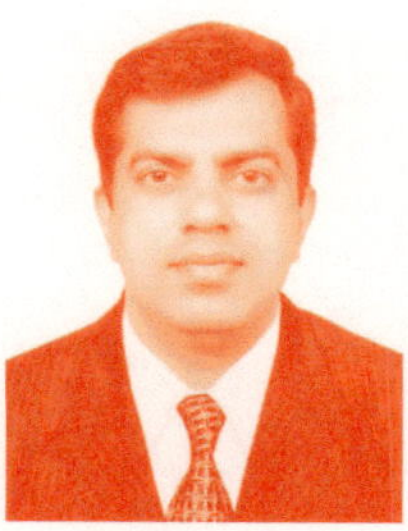
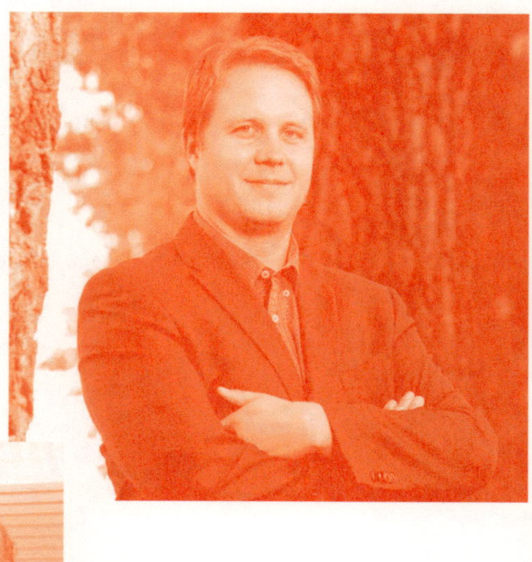
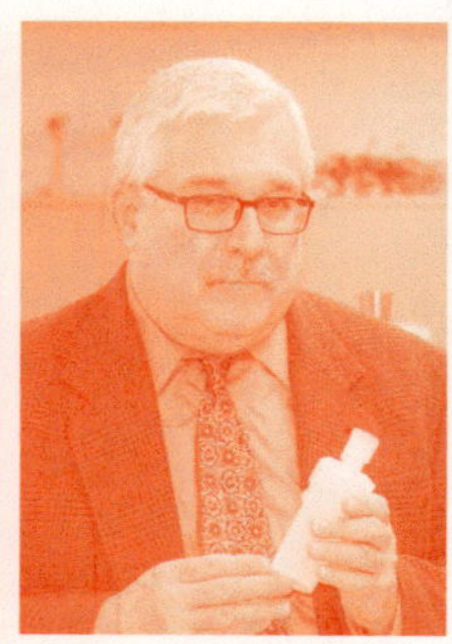
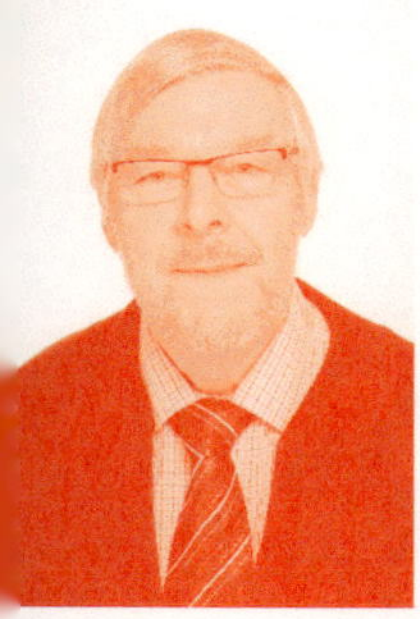
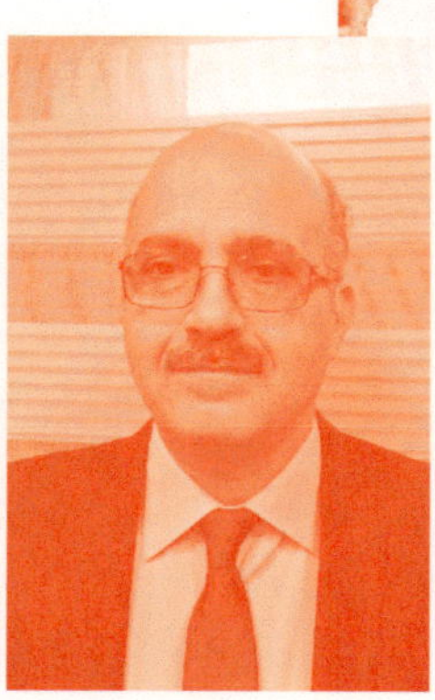
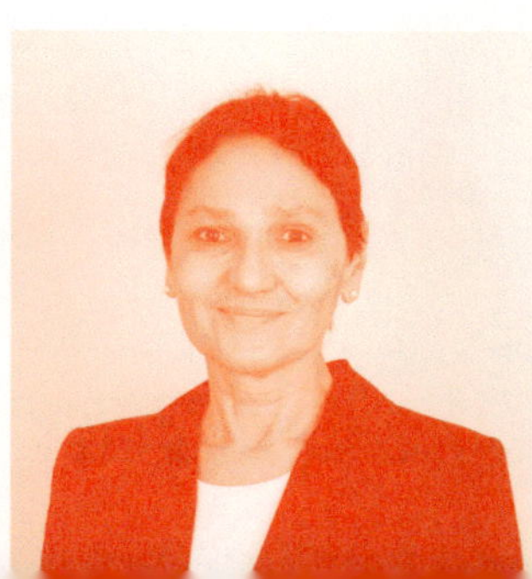
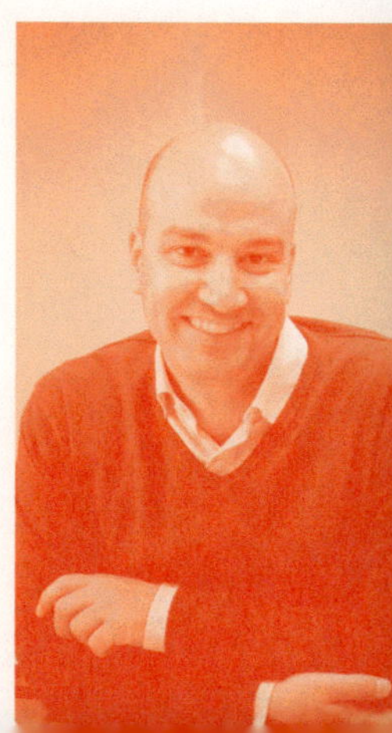

Recent Advances in Laparoscopic Surgery
http://dx.doi.org/10.5772/intechopen.78455
Edited by Francisco M. Sánchez Margallo and Juan A. Sánchez-Margallo

Contributors
José Anacleto Dutra De Resende Júnior, Rodrigo Ribeiro Vieiralves, Renata Teles Buere, Claudio Peixoto Crispi, Makoto Hashizume, Ryu Nakadate, Rafael Gutiérrez Horrillo, Kostas Gianikellis, Miguel Rodal, Francisco Miguel Sánchez-Margallo, Jesus Usón-Gargallo, Juan Alberto Sánchez Margallo, Suzanne Rebecca Pruijssers, Nicole Bouvy, Hytham Hamid, Sean M. Johnston

First published in London, United Kingdom, 2019 by IntechOpen
IntechOpen is the global imprint of INTECHOPEN LIMITED, registered in England and Wales, registration number: 11086078, 7th floor, 10 Lower Thames Street, London, EC3R 6AF, United Kingdom
Printed in Croatia

British Library Cataloguing-in-Publication Data
A catalogue record for this book is available from the British Library

Additional hard and PDF copies can be obtained from orders@intechopen.com

Recent Advances in Laparoscopic Surgery
Edited by Francisco M. Sánchez Margallo and Juan A. Sánchez-Margallo
p. cm.
Print ISBN 978-1-83962-584-8
Online ISBN 978-1-83962-586-2
eBook (PDF) ISBN 978-1-83962-585-5

For EU product safety concerns:
IN TECH d.o.o., Prolaz Marije Krucifikse Kozulić 3, 51000 Rijeka, Croatia, info@intechopen.com or visit our website at intechopen.com.

Meet the editors

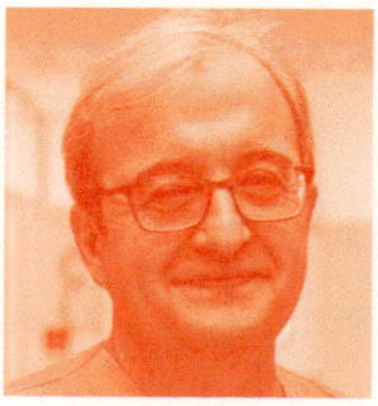

Francisco M. Sánchez-Margallo is the scientific director of the Jesus Usón Minimally Invasive Surgery Centre (JUMISC) in Cáceres (Spain), director of the affiliated Centre of the University of Extremadura, and the deputy director of the Spanish Scientific and Technical Infrastructure (Nanbiosis). His focus is on surgical training and translational research, as well as innovation and technology transfer in the fields of minimally invasive surgery and general healthcare. He has led and participated in European and national research projects related to surgery, medical technology, and imaging diagnosis in laparoscopic and endoscopic procedures, among others. He is director and lecturer of several official master's degrees, has led and taught training residencies, and has conducted doctoral theses of specialists in the health sciences.

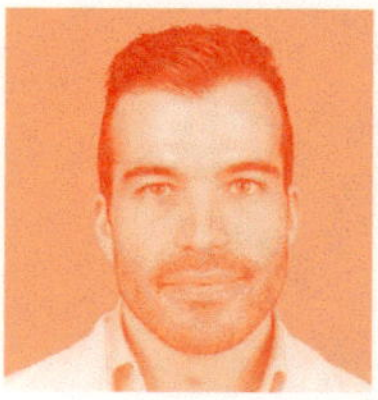

Juan A. Sánchez Margallo is a research scientist at the Bioengineering and Health Technology Unit of the Jesús Usón Minimally Invasive Surgery Centre (Spain). He obtained his PhD degree with European Mention from the University of Extremadura within the field of Bioengineering, obtaining a PhD Extraordinary Award. He did a postdoctoral specialization at the Department of Medical Technology of SINTEF Technology and Society (Norway) and the Department of Biomechanical Engineering, Technical University of Delft (the Netherlands). He has participated in several R&D projects funded by European, national, and regional competitive programs related to medical technology.

Contents

Preface **XI**

Section 1
Introduction and Basic Aspects of Minimally Invasive Surgery **1**

Chapter 1 **3**
Introductory Chapter: Addressing the Challenges of Laparoscopic Surgery
by Francisco M. Sánchez-Margallo, Juan A. Sánchez-Margallo and Jesús Usón

Chapter 2 **9**
Advanced Ergonomics in Laparoscopic Surgery
by Kostas Gianikellis, Andreas Skiadopoulos, Rafael Gutiérrez Horrillo, Miguel Rodal, Juan Alberto Sánchez-Margallo and Francisco M. Sánchez-Margallo

Section 2
Gastrointestinal Surgery **33**

Chapter 3 **35**
Endoluminal Techniques to Treat Obesity
by Suzanne Pruijssers, Ernst van Heurn and Nicole Bouvy

Chapter 4 **55**
LaparoEndoscopic Single-Site Upper Gastrointestinal Surgery
by Hytham K.S. Hamid and Sean M. Johnston

Section 3
Endometriosis Surgery **73**

Chapter 5 **75**
New Paradigms in Endometriosis Surgery of the Distal Ureter
by José Anacleto Dutra de Resende Júnior, Rodrigo Ribeiro Vieiralves, Renata Teles Buere and Claudio Peixoto Crispi

Section 4
Robotic Surgery **91**

Chapter 6 **93**
Intelligent Information-Guided Robotic Surgery
by Ryu Nakadate and Makoto Hashizume

Preface

Minimally invasive surgery has led to a paradigm shift in surgical techniques over the past thirty years. Open surgical procedures are gradually being replaced with minimally invasive methods. In recent times, we have witnessed the development of different technological advances in surgery, new surgical approaches, and the introduction of surgical robotics in daily clinical practice. This technology along with highly skilled work by surgeons have allowed the laparoscopic approach to be applied in a wide range of surgical procedures across all medical specialties.

Technology is an essential part of our everyday lives, and medicine and surgery have also adopted some current technological advances to benefit patients. Everything seems to indicate that the future of surgery will remain closely linked to robotics, image-assisted surgery, wearable technologies, and others, such as artificial intelligence, that are still evolving. However, it will be a while before we know their true impact on clinical medicine.

Aimed at surgeons of all levels, this book outlines some of the most recent advances in the field of laparoscopic surgery. We have collected valuable contributions from relevant surgeons who present their diagnostic and therapeutic experience using minimally invasive approaches. Topics range from surgical robotics to the use of the transanal approach and single-incision laparoscopic surgery, among others.

We hope you enjoy reading this book as much as we enjoyed preparing it.

Francisco M. Sánchez Margallo and Juan A. Sánchez-Margallo
Jesús Usón Minimally Invasive Surgery Centre,
Cáceres, Spain

Section 1

Introduction and Basic Aspects of Minimally Invasive Surgery

Chapter 1

Introductory Chapter: Addressing the Challenges of Laparoscopic Surgery

Francisco M. Sánchez-Margallo, Juan A. Sánchez-Margallo and Jesús Usón

1. Introduction

The field of surgery has experienced a revolution in the present era with a dramatic shift from the traditional open surgery to minimally invasive surgery (MIS). This has been associated to numerous advantages over open surgery, mainly for patients, such as a reduction of tissue trauma and smaller postoperative scars, which in turn involves shorter hospital stays, reduction of the postoperative pain, and faster recovery.

Apart from all these meaningful benefits, this evolution in surgery also results in many technical challenges for surgeons. Relative to open surgery, surgeons lose direct vision, and only two-dimensional indirect vision through a display is available. This indirect vision sometimes takes the sense of orientation and depth perception away from surgeons. The precise manipulation of the laparoscopic instrument tip is restricted mainly because these instruments are generally slim and long and with limited dexterity. Most of the instruments are straight and do not have flexible tips. This surgical tools also lead to a reduction of sensory feedback during surgery due to surgeons cannot directly touch the organs in the body. Some of these limitations make the development of common surgical procedures in open surgery not as straightforward and simple through minimally invasive surgery.

This book is just a step forward for the readers to learn further the recent surgical techniques and technologies that have emerged in order to deal with the aforementioned challenges in minimally invasive surgery.

Laparoscopic surgeons are required long training time, experience, and practices in order to deal with the technical limitations introduced by laparoscopic surgery and become proficient. Due to the steep learning curve that laparoscopic surgery demands in certain surgical procedures, advanced and structured training programs and methods are constantly being introduced [1, 2]. Recently, there is a paradigm shift from traditional subjective assessment methods of trainees to more objective assessment tools that can accredit surgeons as competent in laparoscopic surgery [3, 4].

Despite the many advantages laparoscopic surgery offers to patients, laparoscopy also entails a number of technical limitations for surgeons. The performance of this surgical technique implies important restrictions on freedom of movement, mainly due to the use of rigid and long surgical instruments with poor ergonomic design, the location of the screens, the use of pedals to control the diathermy system, and by the fixed surgical ports for the instruments. These limitations result in an increased incidence of static postures in surgeons and the adoption and maintenance of forced body postures for long periods of time, which potentially affect performance and accuracy during surgery and increase the incidence of physical fatigue and musculoskeletal disorders. In order to address some of these technical limitations, new surgical instruments and devices have been developed aiming to enhance the dexterity, accuracy, and ergonomics of laparoscopic instruments [5]. In addition, new methodological approaches and instrumental techniques for ergonomic analysis have been implemented to improve the working conditions of surgeons, as well as the design of the laparoscopic material [6].

Since the introduction of laparoscopic surgery several decades ago, it has been constantly evolving to the emergence of more sophisticated approaches such as the laparoendoscopic single-site surgery (LESS), natural orifice transluminal endoscopic surgery (NOTES), or transanal surgery, which are intended to reduce the patient's invasiveness and surgical outcomes.

LESS surgery could possibly result in even better postoperative outcomes than multi-port laparoscopic surgery, especially concerning cosmetic outcomes and pain [7, 8]. By reducing the number of transcutaneous points of access, the approach offers numerous advantages including, but not limited to, improving postoperative recovery time and pain, enhancing cosmetics, and minimizing port-related complications. Instrument collision, lack of triangulation, and in-line vision are among the main challenges of LESS surgery. Several techniques and advancements have been introduced to overcome constraints associated with this surgical approach such as novel access devices and curved, articulated, or pre-bent instruments [9, 10]. The feasibility of LESS for almost all types of upper gastrointestinal procedures has been proved [11, 12].

To date, several NOTES procedures have been performed using mainly stomach, rectum, and vagina as the portal of entry into the peritoneal cavity. The main benefits of this surgical technique in comparison to conventional laparoscopic surgery include no scars, less external pain, and lower cost. However, there are also some barriers when using this technique, some of them include difficulty in the closure of enterectomy, anastomotic techniques, spatial orientation, long learning curve, lack of triangulation of instruments, control of hemorrhage, and prevention of the transluminal spread of infection [13]. In order to address some of these technical difficulties in NOTES surgery, novel devices and robotic platforms using a flexible endoscope are appearing as a new trend in the field of MIS [14, 15].

Rectal cancer surgery has undergone a rapid change over the last few decades. We have come a long way from abdominoperineal resection to minimally invasive sphincter-preserving techniques. Minimally invasive surgical techniques have been applied to rectal surgery for several procedures such as transanal polyp excision, local excision of rectal cancer, or transanal total mesorectal excision (taTME), among others [16, 17]. Currently, the two most popular options for local excision are transanal endoscopic microsurgery (TEM) and transanal minimally invasive surgery (TAMIS) [18, 19]. TEM utilizes a rigid platform to access intraluminal lesions in the rectum, maintaining stable the pneumoperitoneum. TAMIS utilizes conventional laparoscopic devices and a single incision port rather than a specialized platform.

One of the technological fields that has most recently affected laparoscopic surgery is robotics. Robotic surgery is a further advancement in the field of laparoscopic surgery, which has gained global acceptance, and a large number of centers are performing robotic surgery as a routine. Laparoscopic robotic surgery has made tremendous progress in a relatively short period of time, resulting in improvements for both the patient and surgeon. Generally speaking, the robot for laparoscopic surgery provides three-dimensional vision, dexterity, and intuitiveness. The majority of robotic surgery applications are in urology, gynecology, and colorectal application, providing comparable clinical results to conventional laparoscopic approaches for the most popular procedures in these fields [20, 21]. The da Vinci surgical system is the most extended robotic platform worldwide for laparoscopic surgery. However, recently many other robotic systems are under development, including additional features such as enhanced portability and force feedback [22, 23].

Author details

Francisco M. Sánchez-Margallo*, Juan A. Sánchez-Margallo and Jesús Usón
Jesús Usón Minimally Invasive Surgery Centre, Cáceres, Spain

*Address all correspondence to: msanchez@ccmijesususon.com

References

[1] Forgione A, Guraya SY. The cutting-edge training modalities and educational platforms for accredited surgical training: A systematic review. Journal of Research in Medical Sciences : The Official Journal of Isfahan University of Medical Sciences. 2017;**22**:51. DOI: 10.4103/jrms.JRMS_809_16

[2] Enciso S, Díaz-Güemes I, Pérez-Medina T, Zapardiel I, de Santiago J, Usón J, et al. Validation of a structured intensive laparoscopic course for basic and advanced gynecologic skills training. International Journal of Gynaecology and Obstetrics. 2016;**133**(2):241-244. DOI: 10.1016/j.ijgo.2015.09.011

[3] Sánchez-Margallo JA, Sánchez-Margallo FM, Oropesa I, Enciso S, Gómez EJ. Objective assessment based on motion-related metrics and technical performance in laparoscopic suturing. International Journal of Computer Assisted Radiology and Surgery. 2017;**12**:307-314. DOI: 10.1007/s11548-016-1459-3

[4] Pérez-Escamirosa F, Chousleb-Kalach A, Hernández-Baro M del C, Sánchez-Margallo JA, Lorias-Espinoza D, Minor-Martínez A. Construct validity of a video-tracking system based on orthogonal cameras approach for objective assessment of laparoscopic skills. International Journal of Computer Assisted Radiology and Surgery 2016;**11**:2283-2293. DOI: 10.1007/s11548-016-1388-1

[5] Sánchez-Margallo JA, Sánchez-Margallo FM. Initial experience using a robotic-driven laparoscopic needle holder with ergonomic handle: Assessment of surgeons' task performance and ergonomics. International Journal of Computer Assisted Radiology and Surgery. 2017;**12**:2069-2077. DOI: 10.1007/s11548-017-1636-z

[6] Sánchez-Margallo FM, Sánchez-Margallo JA. Ergonomics in laparoscopic surgery. In: Malik AM, editor. Laparoscopic Surgery. London: InTech; 2017. pp. 105-123

[7] Evans L, Manley K. Is there a cosmetic advantage to single-incision laparoscopic surgical techniques over standard laparoscopic surgery? A systematic review and meta-analysis. Surgical Laparoscopy, Endoscopy & Percutaneous Techniques. 2016;**26**(3):177-182. DOI: 10.1097/SLE.0000000000000261

[8] Marks JH, Montenegro GA, Shields MV, Frenkel JL, Marks GJ. Single-port laparoscopic colorectal surgery shows equivalent or better outcomes to standard laparoscopic surgery: Results of a 190-patient, 7-criterion case-match study. Surgical Endoscopy. 2015;**29**(6):1492-1499. DOI: 10.1007/s00464-014-3830-1

[9] Sánchez-Margallo FM, Sánchez-Margallo JA. Assessment of postural ergonomics and surgical performance in laparoendoscopic single-site surgery using a handheld robotic device. Surgical Innovation. 2018;**25**:208-217. DOI: 10.1177/1553350618759768

[10] Matos-Azevedo AM, Díaz-Guëmes Martín-Portugués I, Pérez-Duarte FJ, Sánchez-Hurtado MÁ, Sánchez-Margallo FM. Comparison of single access devices during cut and suturing tasks on simulator. The Journal of Surgical Research. 2014;**192**:356-367. DOI: 10.1016/j.jss.2014.06.017

[11] Lee CM, Park DW, Jung DH, Jang YJ, Kim JH, Park S, et al. Single-port laparoscopic proximal gastrectomy with double tract reconstruction for early gastric cancer: Report of a case. Journal of Gastric Cancer. 2016;**16**:200-206. DOI: 10.5230/jgc.2016.16.3.200

[12] Machado MA, Surjan RC, Makdissi FF. Laparoscopic distal pancreatectomy using single-port platform: Technique, safety, and feasibility in a clinical case series. Journal of Laparoendoscopic & Advanced Surgical Techniques. Part A. 2015;**25**(7):581-585. DOI: 10.1089/lap.2015.0032

[13] Rattner D, Kalloo A, ASGE/SAGES Working Group. ASGE/SAGES Working Group on natural orifice translumenal endoscopic surgery, October 2005. Surgical Endoscopy. 2006;**20**(2):329-333

[14] Okamoto Y, Nakadate R, Nakamura S, Arata J, Oguri S, Moriyama T, et al. Colorectal endoscopic submucosal dissection using novel articulating devices: A comparative study in a live porcine model. Surgical Endoscopy. 2018. DOI: 10.1007/s00464-018-6408-5 [Epub ahead of print]

[15] Légner A, Diana M, Halvax P, Liu Y-Y, Zorn L, Zanne P, et al. Endoluminal surgical triangulation 2.0: A new flexible surgical robot. Preliminary pre-clinical results with colonic submucosal dissection. International Journal of Medical Robotics. 2017;**13**:e1819. DOI: 10.1002/rcs.1819

[16] Erkan A, Kelly JJ, Monson JRT. Current state of transanal minimally invasive surgery in the management of rectal cancer. Mini-invasive Surgery. 2018;**2**:30. DOI: 10.20517/2574-1225.2018.51

[17] Penna M, Hompes R, Arnold S, Wynn G, Austin R, Warusavitarne J, et al. Transanal total mesorectal excision: International registry results of the first 720 cases. Annals of Surgery. 2017;**266**(1):111-117. DOI: 10.1097/SLA.0000000000001948

[18] Keller DS, Tahilramani RN, Flores-Gonzalez JR, Mahmood A, Haas EM. Transanal minimally invasive surgery: Review of indications and outcomes from 75 consecutive patients. Journal of the American College of Surgeons. 2016;**222**(5):814-822. DOI: 10.1016/j.jamcollsurg.2016.02.003

[19] Saclarides TJ. Transanal endoscopic microsurgery. Clinics in Colon and Rectal Surgery. 2015;**28**(3):165-175. DOI: 10.1055/s-0035-1562889

[20] Peters BS, Armijo PR, Krause C, Choudhury SA, Oleynikov D. Review of emerging surgical robotic technology. Surgical Endoscopy. 2018;**32**:1636-1655. DOI: 10.1007/s00464-018-6079-2

[21] Szold A, Bergamaschi R, Broeders I, Dankelman J, Forgione A, Langø T, et al. European Association of Endoscopic Surgeons (EAES) consensus statement on the use of robotics in general surgery. Surgical Endoscopy. 2015;**29**(2):253-288. DOI: 10.1007/s00464-014-3916-9

[22] Gueli Alletti S, Perrone E, Cianci S, Rossitto C, Monterossi G, Bernardini F, et al. 3 mm Senhance robotic hysterectomy: A step towards future perspectives. Journal of Robotic Surgery. 2018;**12**:575-577. DOI: 10.1007/s11701-018-0778-5

[23] Hagn U, Konietschke R, Tobergte A, Nickl M, Jörg S, Kübler B, et al. DLR MiroSurge: A versatile system for research in endoscopic telesurgery. International Journal of Computer Assisted Radiology and Surgery. 2010;**5**:183-193. DOI: 10.1007/s11548-009-0372-4

Chapter 2

Advanced Ergonomics in Laparoscopic Surgery

Kostas Gianikellis, Andreas Skiadopoulos, Rafael Gutiérrez Horrillo, Miguel Rodal, Juan Alberto Sánchez-Margallo and Francisco M. Sánchez-Margallo

Abstract

Applied ergonomics is very important in minimally invasive surgery (MIS), especially with the introduction of robotized techniques that have changed the surgeons' work conditions. However, the main aim remains the engineering to enable the compatibility of fulfillment of surgeons' tasks in a physical, logical, and organizational environment with security, comfort, and efficiency. Ergonomics contribution is oriented both to design and redesign utilized material and to work organization. Epidemiological studies have shown the appearance of musculoskeletal pathologies in surgeons performing MIS; therefore, it is relevant to identify the intensity, frequency, and duration of risk factors (posture, repeatability, level of effort, touch pressure, and vibration if relevant) associated with this profession. A further relevant consequence of the effort applied during MIS is local muscle fatigue (LMF), an important factor to consider in musculoskeletal pathologies. The aim of this chapter is to present different methodological approaches by employing most advanced technologies to define the most appropriate posture that surgeons should adopt during MIS to decrease LMF apparition risk level and at the same time to increase capacity to variate the posture without reducing the precision task performance.

Keywords: laparoscopy, ergonomics, musculoskeletal disorders

1. Introduction

Ergonomics can be defined as an interdisciplinary field of knowledge to study the characteristics, needs, and abilities of human beings, analyzing those aspects that affect the design of products and/or production processes. In all the applications, its objective is to try to adapt products, tasks, tools, spaces, and the environment in general to the biological characteristics, the capabilities, and the needs of the people in order to guarantee the safety and health of workers, users, and consumers as well as to increase their welfare and improve the production processes' efficiency [1].

Laparoscopic surgery as a technique of minimally invasive surgery began to be applied in the early 1990s and refers to surgical operations in the abdomen or pelvic cavity. Although this technique is very advantageous for the patient in comparison with an "open" surgical intervention [2], it is a technically challenging one for the surgeon [3, 4].

On the other hand, the "**fine handling**" associated with the performance of laparoscopic surgery techniques, related to very low frequency and relatively small amplitude motor patterns as movements are restricted due to the fixed holes through which the laparoscopic instruments are introduced, implies maintenance of the posture during relatively long intervals of time along with high levels of musculoskeletal effort and lack of comfort sensation.

Scientific studies have shown that the use of laparoscopic instruments contributes to significantly increase the activity of the deltoid muscle and at the same time the activity of the superficial flexor and common extensor digitorum [5, 6], promoting the appearance of local muscle fatigue in the upper extremities and in the neck area as well as numbness in the fingers [7–12].

To the aforementioned, it should be added that the minimally invasive surgery techniques also involve control of the position and orientation of the trunk and head, the segments whose mass is relatively large, reaching almost 50% of the total body and therefore involving a high muscular effort during relatively long time intervals. In addition, surgeons have to manipulate instruments that are not designed with ergonomic usability criteria, since the level of force and contact pressure implied by their use (clamp and grip) are unknown. Finally, the use of monitors during surgical operations implies an additional difficulty for surgeons as there is no tactile interaction with the organs undergoing the operation [13, 14].

In this scenario, it is very common to adopt and maintain awkward postures for relatively long periods of time, which cause a high level of physical load associated with the intervention of the muscles that control the involved joints of the locomotor system. These factors can cause discomfort and musculoskeletal pain or even disorders that can lead to permanent disability and/or need for surgical intervention (**Figure 1**).

This type of pathology develops progressively in **stages**, so that in the first stage, moderate fatigue and initial discomfort that are usually moderate are observed. In the second stage, there are occasional discomforts in the posture and mild pain that disappears with a good rest. Then, as a consequence of the continued exposure to the risk factors, pain and other symptoms that persist almost throughout the day appear causing a process of progressive degradation that leads to more severe pain

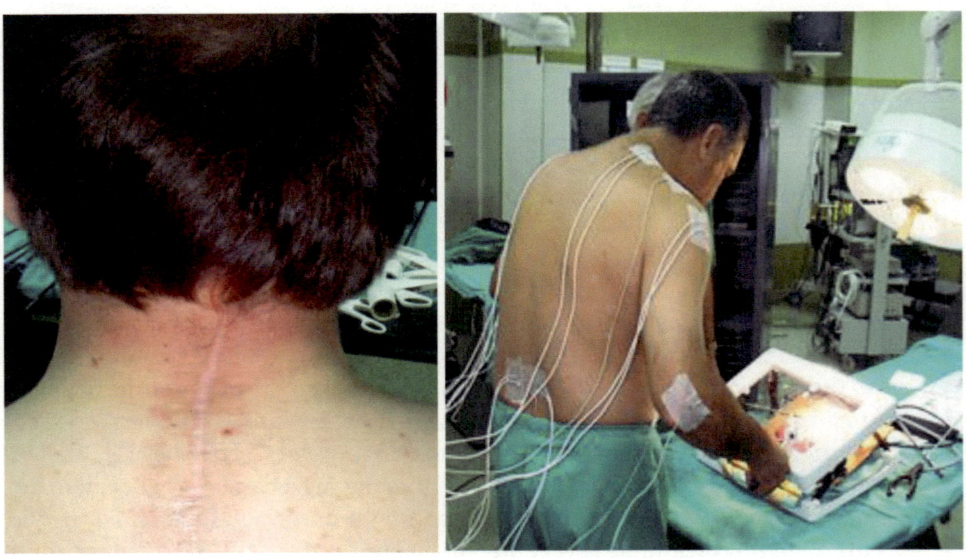

Figure 1.
Neck surgery (left) and Surgery training (right).

and ends up compromising the daily activity. This ends in a chronic disability that reduces the normal physical abilities of the person and seriously affects his/her quality of daily life.

Since two decades, the European Agency for Safety and Health at Work [15], at the request of the European Commission, has issued two reports on musculoskeletal disorders and injuries related to work. In these reports, the social and economic dimension of musculoskeletal pathologies has been confirmed as well as the need to establish standardized scientific criteria for the evaluation of their risk factors. Secondly, the reliability of the epidemiological data is questioned and the reconsideration of experimental studies is recommended as there is no consensus on the confirmation of the appearance of local muscle fatigue as a risk factor in association with the adoption of forced working postures and the performance of repetitive movements. In this sense, ergonomic intervention based on scientific work is recommended for the development of strategies for the evaluation and prevention of risk factors for musculoskeletal pathologies.

The objective of this chapter is, starting with the results of an epidemiological study (Nordic Questionnaire), to present the results of the research work carried out by the collaboration between the Jesús Usón Minimally Invasive Surgery Centre and the BioẼrgon research group during the last 15 years based on the methodology of ergonomics and using the instrumental techniques of Biomechanics of Human Movement to contribute to investigate the level of physical effort borne by surgeons and to establish ergonomic criteria to improve the working conditions of surgeons, as well as to establish ergonomic design criteria for laparoscopic material by analyzing different tasks in laparoscopic surgery in conjunction with the motor behavior of surgeons.

In this sense, the results of the research are useful to manage organizational and ergonomic decision-making with the aim of introducing an ergonomic conception of laparoscopic surgery processes to improve surgeons' occupational health and quality of life. The application of these measures requires to previously identify and evaluate the risk factors. This means to select the tasks and jobs with exposure to risk of injury, to study which is the level of exposure in each of them, and to decide in which cases it is necessary to apply correction measures.

The possibilities offered by **Biomechanics** to raise and solve problems related to the improvement of health and quality of life have consolidated it as a field of knowledge in continuous expansion, capable of providing scientific and technological solutions. On the other hand, the industrial projection of Biomechanics has reached several sectors, providing the basis for the conception and adaptation of numerous products, for diagnostic techniques and for the evaluation of human motor skills.

The objective of the applied research in the occupational field is to analyze working conditions, especially the interface "man-workplace" or "man-machine" as a way to prevent discomfort and/or occupational pathologies, to reduce fatigue and increase the comfort and to generate criteria for the design of tools and jobs according to the characteristics of the users and the tasks to be performed.

2. Epidemiology study

The epidemiological study enables collection of data regarding the incidence of musculoskeletal pathologies in laparoscopic surgery and the risk factors, which favor their appearance [16].

The study was conducted on a sample of 52 surgeons (35–65 years), (7.31 ± 3.30 years of experience) in the techniques of laparoscopic surgery and (12.9 ± 6.7) hours per week dedicated to them.

The standardized Nordic Musculoskeletal Questionnaire (NMQ) modified by the Health and Safety Executive (HSE) of the United Kingdom was used (**Figure 2**) [17, 18]. The epidemiological study also included the procedure of the National Institute of Health and Safety at Work of the USA [19], which allows to identify the musculoskeletal disorders, the conditions which cause them, as well as the perception of the workers.

According to results of the study, 58% of the survey respondents have suffered **neck** pain (43% in the last 12 months) and 66% attribute it to their activity at work. The frequency of pain in the neck area is high (**Figure 2**). Occasionally, pain is intense to very intense, though in most cases, it is of lower intensity (**Figure 3**).

Thirty-seven percent of the survey respondents have suffered from **shoulder** pain (33% in the last 12 months) and 75% associate it with their activity at work. The frequency of shoulder pain is high with approximately 50% of the subjects reporting intense to very intense pain and with the remaining subjects reporting pain of lower intensity (**Figure 4**).

As regards the **back**, 42% of subjects have suffered pain or discomfort in the upper part (21% in the upper part and 35% in the lower part in the last 12 months); 71% of the survey respondents attribute their back pain to activity at work and 19% have even missed work for this reason. Pathologies of the back occur with a considerably high frequency (**Figure 5**).

Thirty-seven percent of subjects have suffered from pain in the **wrists** and **hands** (31% in the last 12 months). Although the frequency is considerably low (**Figure 6**), 17% have suffered from pain in these areas at least once a month. Although they did not miss work, 6% of survey respondents have seen their work performance affected for at least 1 week due to pain in the wrists and hands.

It is important to highlight the relevance for surgeons of the position they adopt during minimally invasive surgical procedures. In personal interviews, surgeons have stated that the position adopted during surgery is substantial to better perform the intervention (96%), they consider training being necessary in association with the adoption of a comfortable posture during the intervention (88%), and they indicate that they are "forced" to operate by adopting an uncomfortable position according to their subjective perception (46%). The data suggest that the forward inclination of the body is performed unconsciously (67% of respondents). On the other hand, 61% surgeons think that the coordination of the posture

Neck	43%
Low Back	35%
Shoulders	33%
Wrist & Hands	31%
Upper Back	21%
Knees	12%
Elbows	8%
Hips	8%
Ankles	6%

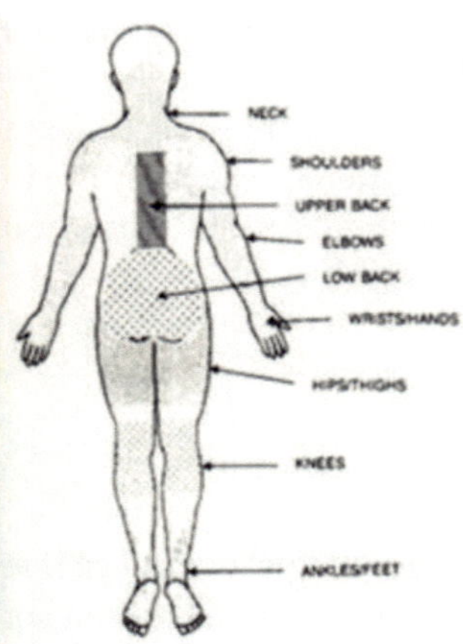

Figure 2.
Anatomical parts of the body analyzed in the epidemiological study and percentage of musculoskeletal discomfort by anatomical regions adapted from [17].

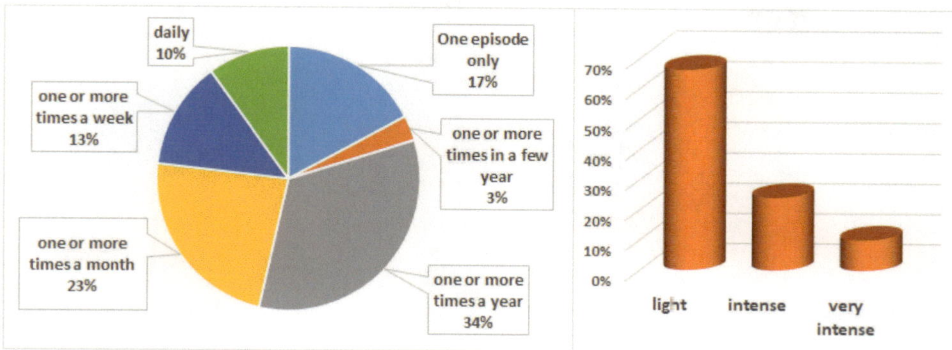

Figure 3.
Frequency of pain appearance and pain intensity in the neck area.

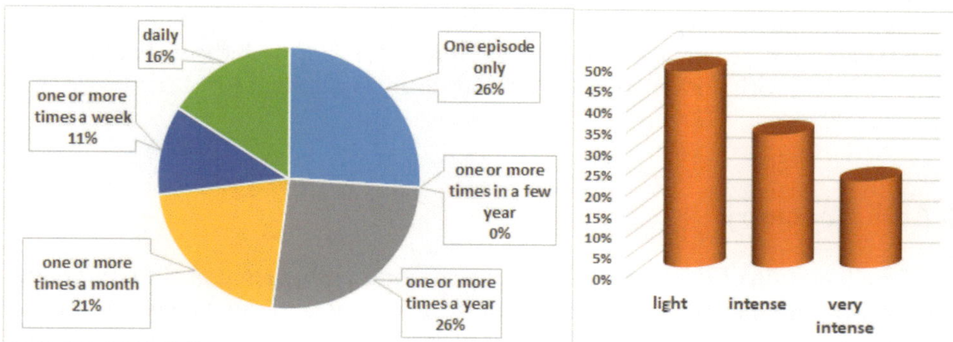

Figure 4.
Frequency of appearance and intensity of shoulder pain.

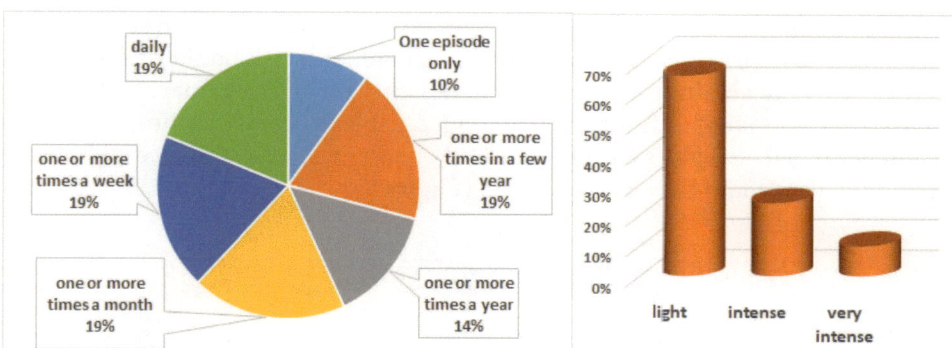

Figure 5.
Frequency of appearance and pain intensity in the back area.

during the surgical procedure appears naturally while for the remaining 39%, it is learned. Furthermore, data suggest that the arrangement of the equipment in the operating room is the cause of the adoption of forced trunk postures (80% of the respondents). These forced postures are due to the distance to the operating table (15%) and due to its height (13%). The placement of the monitor also implies the adoption of an awkward posture (57%). Sixty-two percent of surgeons have problems due to the prolonged maintenance of the posture, 68% indicate the adoption of uncomfortable postures, and 70% indicate the adoption of forced postures. Finally, surgeons were asked about comfort in the use of surgical instruments and

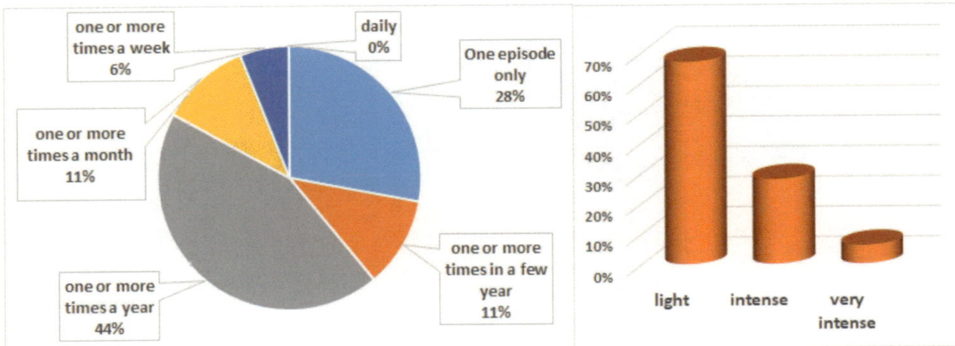

Figure 6.
Frequency of appearance and pain intensity in the wrist-hand area.

they reported having experienced difficulties with handling the needle holder (22%), handling the suction-irrigation equipment (15%), with the view of the monitor (8%), with scissors (6%), with diathermy equipment (6%), and with the dissector (4%).

3. Anthropometry

The adaptation of the laparoscopic surgery's environment and of the equipment based on ergonomic criteria must take into account that the seated position cannot be adopted because it conditions the angle of incidence of the instruments [20] and the morphological characteristics of the users. Anthropometry provides information regarding the dimensions of the human body in a certain (static) position, as well as the ranges of movement of the body parts, reach, trajectories, surfaces, and volumes of movement (functional). Although different types of anthropometers have been developed over the last decades, BioẼrgon Research Group has developed a procedure based on three-dimensional photogrammetry of BiomSoft 2.0 software [21] (**Figure 7**) to obtain anthropometric data assisted by a Vitus Smart XXL® system (human solutions) of full-body scanning, capable to provide anthropometric data in industrial quantities with ±1 mm level of accuracy, in accordance with the international standard DIN EN ISO 20685 (**Figure 8**).

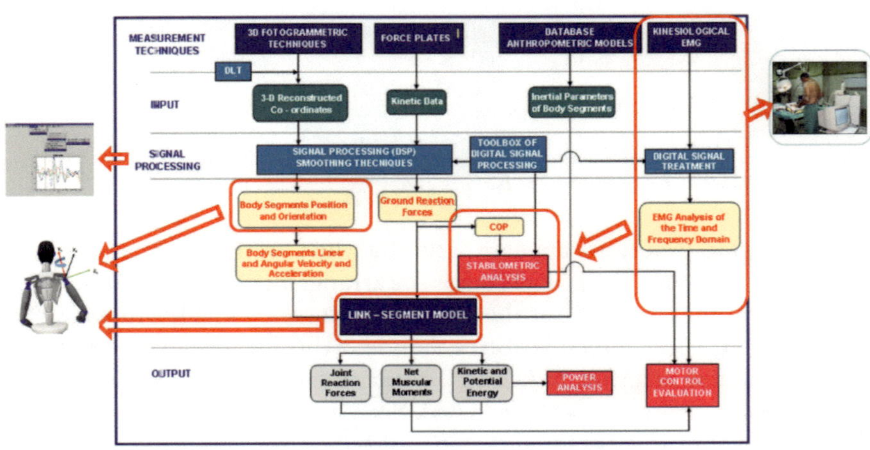

Figure 7.
BiomSoft 2.0 flow chart.

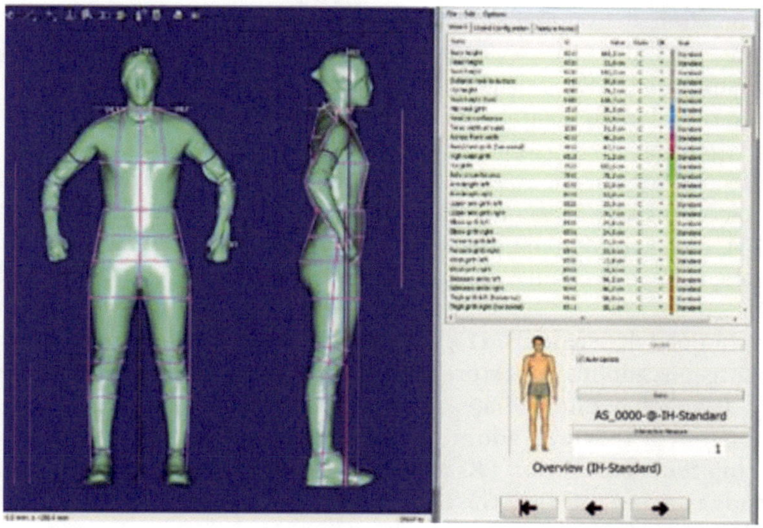

Figure 8.
A 3D scanner for anthropometry.

The obtained information is relevant to formulate criteria and recommendations for ergonomic intervention in the laparoscopic surgery scenario, such as working in a standing position with sufficient space for the hands and with properly dimensioned tools especially in the handles, to avoid tensions in the arm and wrist and to allow handling of the tools to be comfortable for the hands. The ISO 6385 [22] standard recommends adapting the height of the work surface to the user's dimensions for tasks, having enough space for body movements, having tables and controls within reach, and providing tools with handles adapted to the user's hand. The required levels of strength should be within the desirable limits, and the movements of the body should be natural and soft. Finally, the movements of the trunk should not introduce excessive inclinations and/or torsions.

4. Characterization and motor control of posture

4.1 Ovako working posture analysis system

As during the performance of laparoscopic surgery a standing posture is adopted, it is important to regulate and adapt the height of the operating table, the height of the monitor, and its orientation and the space for the feet to be able to operate near the surface of the operating table to the morphological and functional characteristics of the surgeon. The placement of the elements in the surgeon's environment should facilitate the adoption of a comfortable posture, especially in the early stages of learning laparoscopic techniques, avoiding excessive inclinations and/or torsions of the trunk and head, as well as abduction of the shoulders. In this context, characterization studies of the adopted position and its consequences during simulations of laparoscopic operations have been carried out. In the first phase of performed studies, the application of the OWAS protocol [23] was used as a standardized process to characterize the level of risk for tasks and for postures that were forced, nonrepetitive, and without defined work cycles, taking into account the posture of the trunk, arms, and legs as well as depending on the level of the load or force exerted by the surgeon. This process allowed to assess the level of risk for surgeons caused by the maintenance of the analyzed postures for a prolonged period of time. The position of 13 surgeons (four women and nine men) with different levels of experience and specialties was analyzed. The surgeons performed a simulation of a 60-minute laparoscopic surgery at the Jesús Usón Minimally Invasive Surgery Centre, and the adopted position was coded every 20 seconds (**Figure 9**) using a 3D video photogrammetry.

The effective time of the operation was identified as the time during which the subject looks at the screen and handles the surgical instruments with both hands (**Figure 10**). Interruptions could be due to the training process, change in surgical instruments, change in simulation material in the pelvitrainer, and distracting attention.

In the obtained data (**Figure 11**), it can be observed that during the procedures, 12 of the surgeons adopted a posture with **level 2** risk, meaning that intervention is necessary, although not immediate.

The position of this level adopted by a greater number of surgeons sometimes during the intervention (**10 of the surgeons**) was coded as **2121**, which corresponds to a posture with the back inclined, the arms below the shoulder, and standing with both legs straight with a light load ≤10 kg. Furthermore, four surgeons adopted a posture with **level 3** risk of musculoskeletal injuries, implying that the working method should be modified as soon as possible. The posture of this level adopted by a greater number of surgeons sometimes during the intervention was coded as **4231**, which corresponds to a posture with the back bent and turned, one arm above the shoulder, standing with one straight leg, and with a force ≤10 kg. Only one surgeon adopted a posture with a **level 4** risk of musculoskeletal injuries, meaning that corrective measures must be taken immediately.

4.2 3D photogrammetry

As observed previously, it is necessary to use instrumental techniques with a greater discriminatory capacity to characterize the position adopted by surgeons due to the fact that some movements such as bending and rotation of the trunk and head as well as flexion and abduction of the arms have been detected. 3D photogrammetry was utilized in order to quantify the posture of the body segments in 3D. The mechanical model (**Figure 12**) that was used to

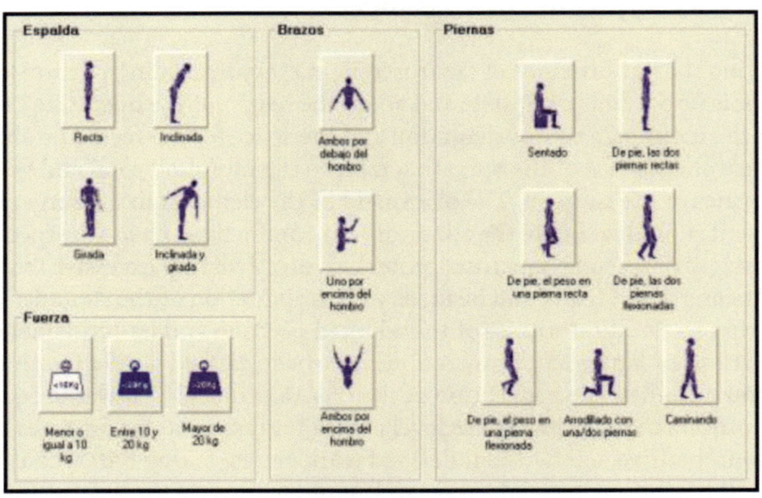

Figure 9.
OWAS protocol (ergo/IBV software®).

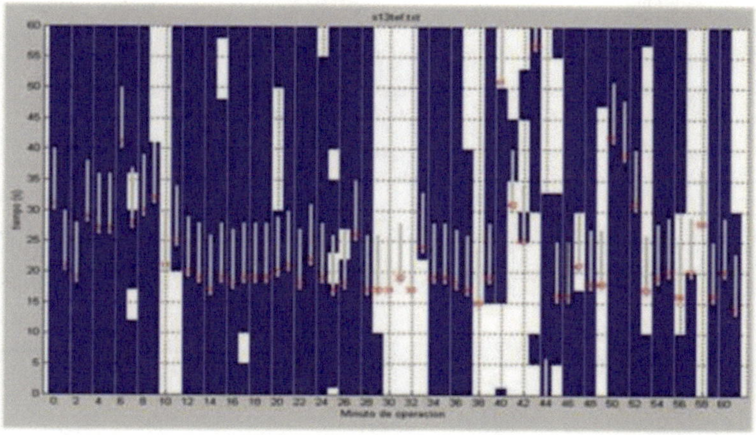

Figure 10.
Recorded surgery time. Blue: effective time and white: EMG record time.

NIVELES DE RIESGO

	POSTURAS									
Subtareas incluidas	Nivel 1		Nivel 2		Nivel 3		Nivel 4		TOTAL	
	Frec.	%	Frec.	%	Frec.	%	Frec.	%	Frec.	%
Sujeto01	124	10.1	8	1.7	0	0.0	0	0.0	132	7.6
Sujeto02	127	10.4	0	0.0	0	0.0	0	0.0	127	7.3
Sujeto03	169	13.8	1	0.2	0	0.0	0	0.0	170	9.8
Sujeto04	96	7.8	20	4.2	0	0.0	0	0.0	116	6.7
Sujeto05	67	5.5	57	12.0	0	0.0	0	0.0	124	7.2
Sujeto06	157	12.8	1	0.2	0	0.0	0	0.0	158	9.1
Sujeto07	47	3.8	93	19.6	0	0.0	0	0.0	140	8.1
Sujeto08	139	11.3	9	1.9	1	2.9	0	0.0	149	8.6
Sujeto09	15	1.2	111	23.4	17	50.0	0	0.0	143	8.2
Sujeto10	21	1.7	117	24.7	2	5.9	1	100.0	141	8.1
Sujeto11	104	8.5	4	0.8	0	0.0	0	0.0	108	6.2
Sujeto12	80	6.5	21	4.4	0	0.0	0	0.0	101	5.8
Sujeto13	79	6.4	32	6.8	14	41.2	0	0.0	125	7.2
TOTAL	1,225	70.6	474	27.3	34	2.0	1	0.1	1,734	100.0

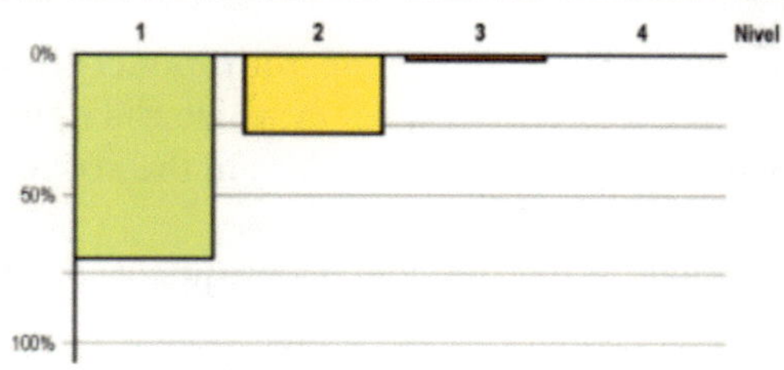

Figure 11.
Report of risk levels.

record the spatial coordinates of the anatomical markers (15 real + 3 virtual) was defined according to the standardized procedures of the kinematic analysis of the International Society of Biomechanics [24]. In this sense, the position was characterized in terms of the Euler angles [25] and the "Joint Coordination System" (JCS) [26], which allow to determine the variation of the orientation of a segment in three dimensions with respect to a local RS. Three markers associated with the monitor and three markers associated with the operating table were added to the mechanical model (**Figure 12**).

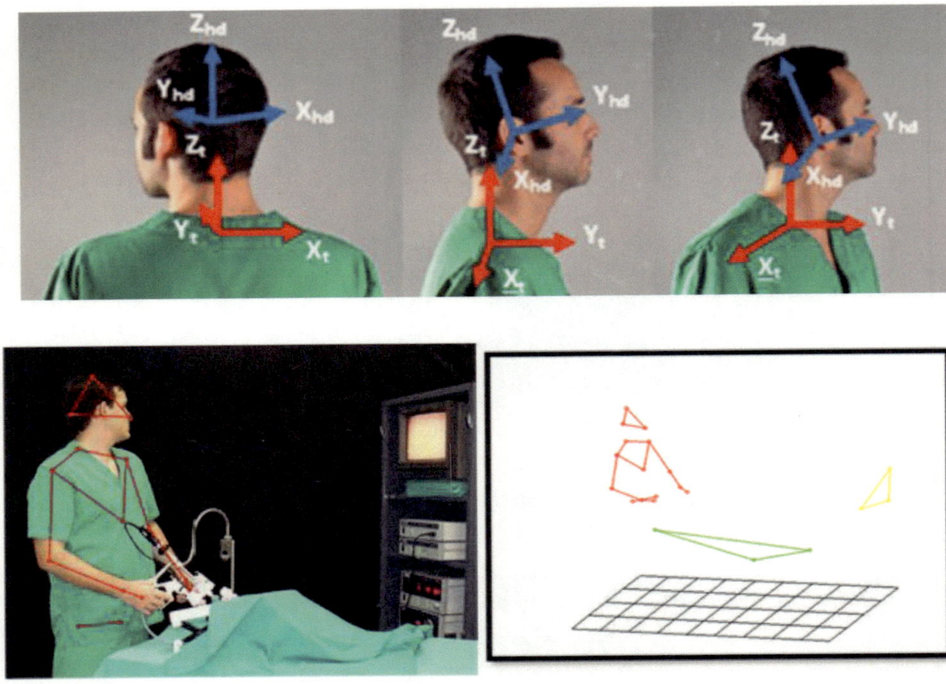

Figure 12.
Mechanical model used for the evaluation of posture by 3D photogrammetry.

The sequence of turns used for the head was Zt-Yh-Xh (**Figure 12**) of the JCS method. Axes are defined as follows:

i. Zt axis of the coordinate system associated with the trunk, which represents the axis with respect to which the flexion (negative)/extension (positive) movement takes place.

ii. Yh axis of the head representing the axis with respect to which the right (negative)/left (positive) rotation movement takes place.

iii. Xh axis has the direction of the "vector product" of the other two axes, representing the axis with respect to which the right (negative)/left (positive) inclination movement takes place in the articulation.

For the body segment of the shoulder, the sequence of turns Yt-Xh-Yh (**Figure 13**) of the Euler angles is as follows:

i. First rotation: the Yt axis of the coordinate system associated with the trunk that represents the axis with respect to which the azimuthal angle takes place (0° is abduction and 90° is forward flexion).

ii. Second rotation: the Xh axis of the humerus that represents the axis with respect to which the lifting movement of the humerus takes place (elevation: positive).

iii. Third rotation: the Yh axis of the humerus that represents the axis with respect to which the internal (positive)/external (negative) rotation movement of the humerus takes place.

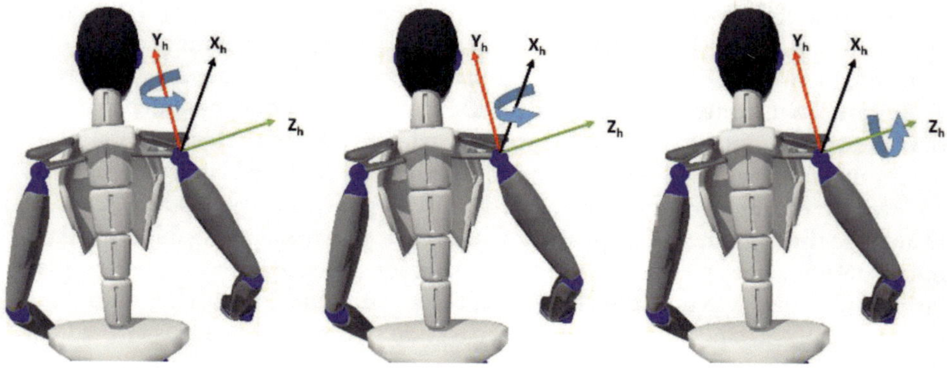

Figure 13.
Definition of the rotations of the right upper limb.

The measurements performed to characterize the position adopted by surgeons during the simulation of laparoscopic operations allowed for the first time to quantify the order of magnitude of the relative orientation of the body segments in laparoscopic surgery. The results obtained on the shoulder joint show that the range of the elevation angle oscillates between 11 and 46.1° with an average of 26.2° ± 7.8 (coeficient of varation (CV) 30%) for the skillful arm, while for the nonskillful arm, it varies between 9.1 and 52.6° with an average of 27.1° ± 10.1 (CV 37%). In both cases, the coefficient of variation is high, a fact that demonstrates the high variability in the position adopted by the surgeons during the surgical procedure as a consequence of the nonexistence of ergonomic criteria for the configuration of the work environment. A high percentage of surgeons operate with an elevation angle close to or greater than 30° associated with the appearance of local muscle fatigue in the shoulder as suggested by other studies [3, 27]; therefore, it is recommended that the range of elevation of the arms is below 30°. The position of the arm is directly related to the height at which the laparoscopic instruments are manipulated. These data suggest adapting the surgical environment to the characteristics of the surgeon taking into account the order of magnitude of the variability found in the studies performed.

As regards the posture of the head, the following values were found: flexion of 14.76° ± 9.86 (CV 67%), extension of 2.8° ± 2.6 (CV 93%), left lateral inclination of 4.75° ± 4.09 (CV 86%), right lateral inclination of 10.71° ± 6.17 (86% CV), internal rotation of 14.21° ± 12.18 (86% CV), and external rotation of 9.31° ± 7.17 (77% CV). The results confirm that the head barely moves (range of motion) as a consequence of the observation of the monitor, and therefore, the muscles that intervene in the maintenance of the posture during relatively long time intervals can experience fatigue [28–30].

As could be seen so far, it is very important to take into account the high variability of the geometric parameters associated with the posture adopted by the analyzed surgeons. Therefore, the question arises whether this variability is "biopositive" or "bionegative" from the point of view of ergonomics and of the prevention of musculoskeletal pathologies of personnel as a consequence of postural and muscular effort.

4.3 Variability study: uncontrolled manifold analysis

As a consequence of what has been described in Section 4.2, it is important to study the variability of the posture in order to test whether variability in upper limbs-joint configuration stabilizes or destabilizes head posture on the sagittal plane as its position is constrained by the displacement of the monitor during conventional laparoscopy (LAP) and Laparoendoscopic Single Site (LESS) surgery approaches. Also, the introduction of a framework to quantify joint coordination and its influence on the posture adopted by surgeons seems to be relevant. Therefore, an uncontrolled manifold (UCM) hypothesis model has been proposed that allows to quantify, globally, kinematic variability in task-relevant and task-irrelevant components and to determine whether the analyzed laparoscopic tasks are performed in healthy ranges or not. The UCM provides a quantitative approach to analyze the influence of imposed constraints, e.g., workplace layout and instruments design on the postural strategy that surgeons choose to accomplish surgical tasks, and it allows to map the variance of three individual joint angles onto the head position variance. Also, it allows separation of the combinations of the mentioned angles that are equally able to stabilize the head position within an acceptable margin of error for those combinations that are irrelevant for the ongoing task (**Figure 14**).

The UCM framework has been used recently to examine whether teleoperation with the da Vinci Si Surgical System manipulator (grip fixture attached to master manipulator) changes the structure of joint variability relative to the freehand (holding the grip fixture alone) in experienced and novice surgeons [31] as well as to analyze whether joint angles cooperate to adjust head position during laparoscopy work [32] (**Figure 15**).

It was shown that the effect of teleoperation on hand movements' stabilization depends on experience and that the head control variable defines an uncontrolled manifold, i.e., joint configurations of upper arm during laparoscopy do not destabilize head position. The motor redundancy, due to the numerous degrees of freedom of the human locomotor apparatus, compared with the substantially lower anatomical constraints that are imposed by the structure of the musculoskeletal system at the level of the joints, gives the surgeons the possibility to adopt an infinite number of postures during work and consequently the ability to execute countless voluntary motor patterns in order to accomplish their tasks.

Eight right-handed experienced surgeons in laparoscopic surgery (>100 laparoscopic procedures) and LESS surgery (>20 procedures using LESS approach) voluntarily accepted to participate in the study. Subjects performed a dissection of the serosa layer on an ex vivo porcine stomach inside a laparoscopic box trainer for

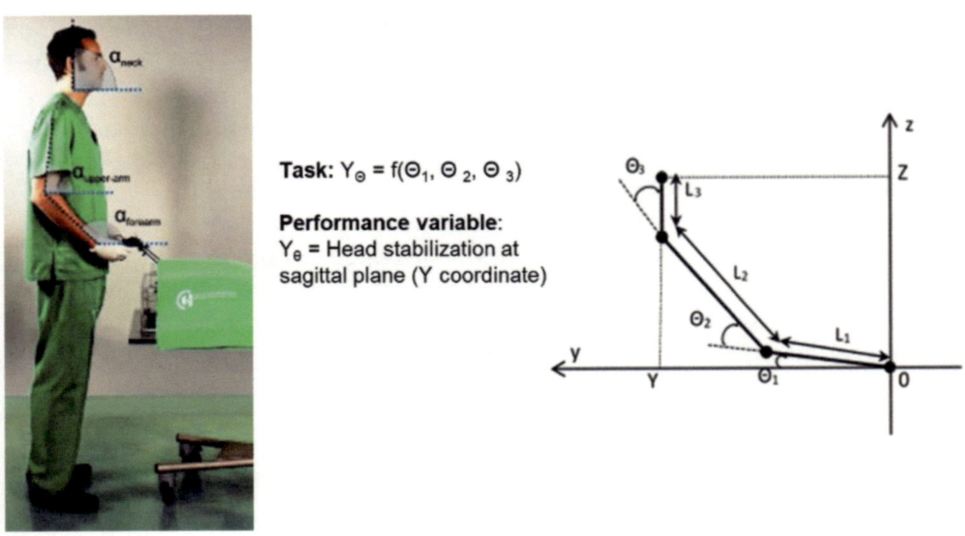

Figure 14.
Mechanical UCM model.

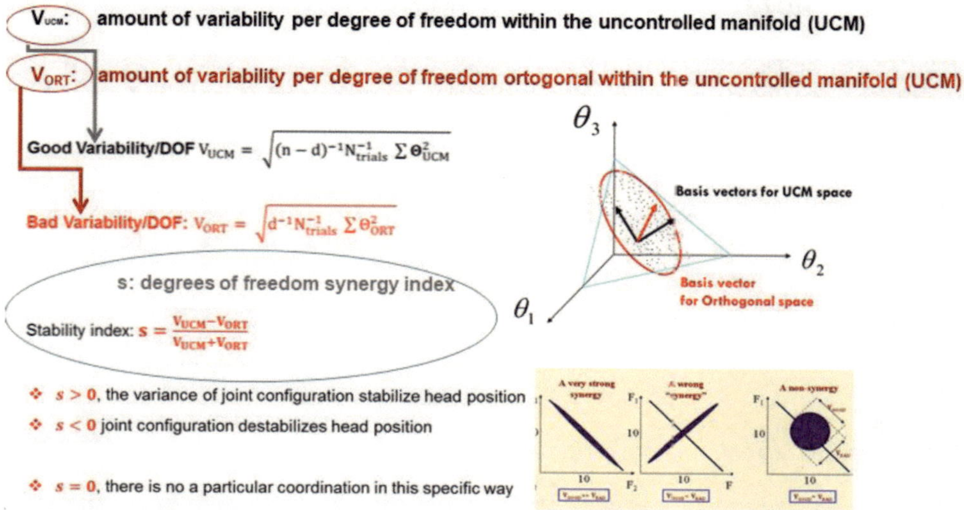

Figure 15.
UCM resume.

10 minutes. This task was carried out by both laparoscopic surgical approach (LAP) and by LESS surgery [33]. A 3D photogrammetry was used to calculate the spatial coordinates of anatomical markers, using the same model as described in Section 4.2. The 3D coordinates of digitized points were obtained using the algorithm known as direct linear transformation (DLT) and were specified with respect to the defined origin of the global reference system. The 3D coordinates were obtained for a total of 40 events (N = 40), an event in every 15 seconds of surgical activity. For the same events, the posture of the head was defined with respect to the trunk, considering posture as the position and orientation of body segments. The trunk and head body segments were defined as solids, and their spatial position and orientation were obtained fixing them to segmental reference frames (SRF). This process allows the measurement of the posture adopted by surgeons in terms of clinically interpreted position and orientation of body segments. The results of the study show that kinematic redundancy enables surgeons to adopt an appropriate posture during surgical tasks, allowing them to avoid uncomfortable postures. However, other constraints other than the anatomical ones may have an impact, in particular joint configurations, i.e., workspace layout and instrumental design. Therefore, the goal of the UCM analysis was to test whether variability in upper-limb joint configuration during two different surgery approaches stabilized or destabilized head posture on the sagittal plane. Although the intertrial variability in joint configuration space should be organized to stabilize manual operation-task movements, by definition, it could also be organized to stabilize other important controlled variables as well. The head posture is a plausible candidate as its position is constrained by the displacement of the monitor. The results of the UCM analysis showed a positive degrees of freedom synergy index indicating that the covariation of the upper-limb joint angles stabilizes the head posture of the surgeons in the anterior-posterior direction. This synergy is stronger in some surgeons (**Figure 16**).

Even though the synergy index takes different values between the LAP and LESS approach (**Figure 17**), there was not a statistically significant difference in the synergy index between the LAP and LESS approach for the UCMs of both the left ($t_{(7)} = 1.76$ and $p = 0.12$) and right joint spaces ($t_{(7)} = 0.127$ and $p = 0.902$). As can be seen in the results of 3D kinematics of the posture of the head with respect to the trunk (**Figure 18**), there is a high variability of the postures adopted by

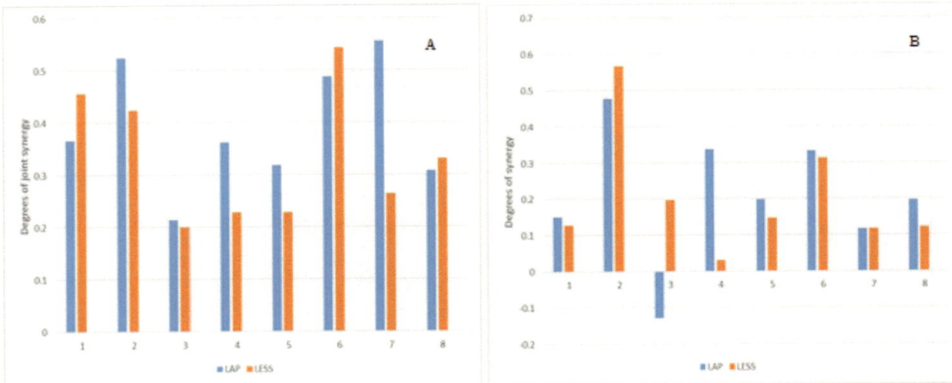

Figure 16.
UCM synergy. (A) Left body side and (B) right body side.

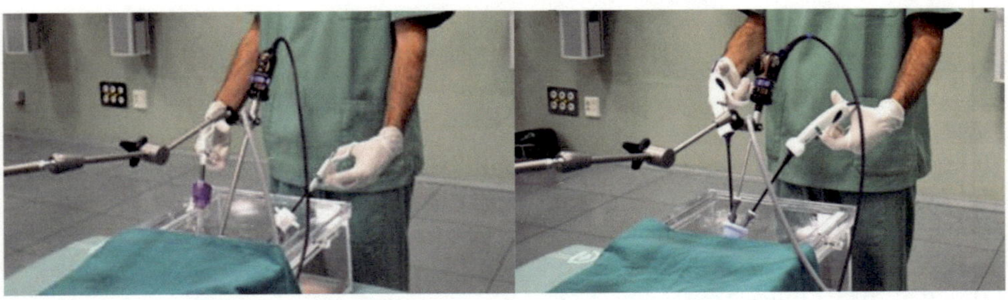

Figure 17.
LAP (left) vs. LESS (right).

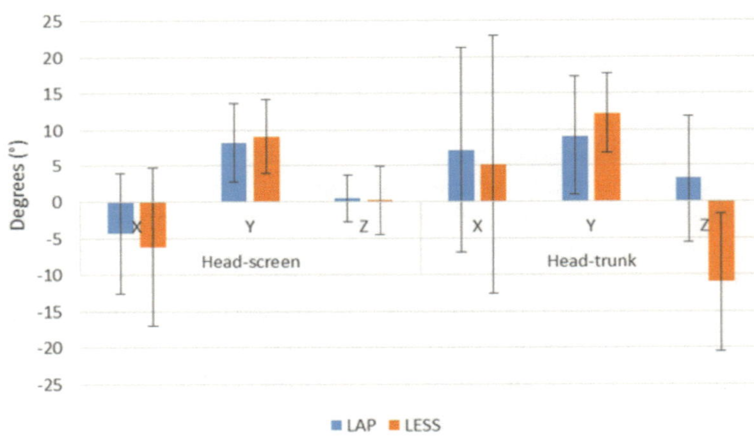

Figure 18.
Results of variability of 3D neck rotation depending on monitor and trunk.

the surgeons. This is due to the fact that surgeons are free to adopt their postures according to their personal judgment. Kinematics of surgeon heads' posture with respect to the trunk indicates high variability because of the adoption of the posture according to the subjective perception. Upper-body joint variability quantified using the framework of the UCM hypothesis allowed to separate the combination of joint angles that were equally able to stabilize mean head posture on sagittal plane for those solutions that destabilized head mean posture.

4.4 Inertial unit measurement system

In the last few years, introduction and use of inertial sensors in the analysis and characterization of posture variability in the context of minimally invasive surgery has been a great advance in biomechanics methodology, as 3D photogrammetry requires a lot of time for digitation of images. This has been the most important reason for BioÈrgon Research group to record and analyze laparoscopic procedures in 3D using this technology, being a pioneer and probably the only one group to use it. Undoubtedly, this is much more an efficient instrumental technique for the characterization of posture in minimally invasive surgery [34]. In this sense, a study using the commercial system XSens MVN Biomech (**Figure 19**) was carried out in the Jesus Usón Minimal Invasive Surgery Center. Eight surgeons participated in the study (four novices and four experts) and performed 24 simple sutures with conventional instruments. The results obtained regarding the position of the surgeons corroborate the high variability found in the studies carried out with 3D photogrammetry. The values found show CV greater than 70% in all joints and especially in the wrist joint flexion-extension and radial and ulnar deviation (**Figure 20**).

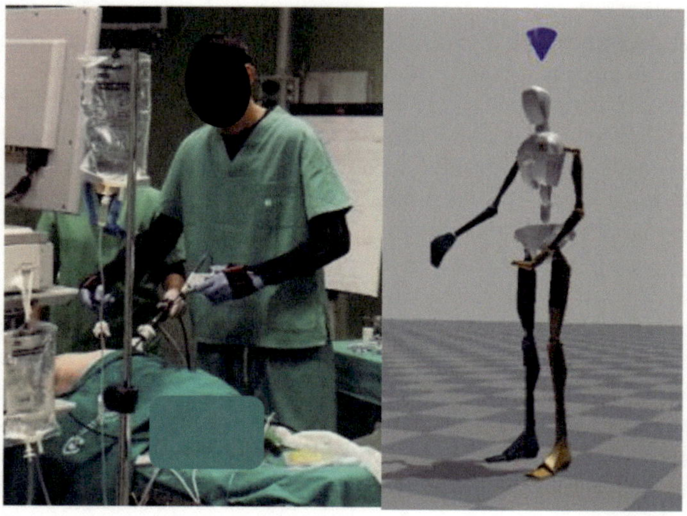

Figure 19.
Sensorized surgeon with inertial measurement units (IMUs) and biomechanical model used by XSens.

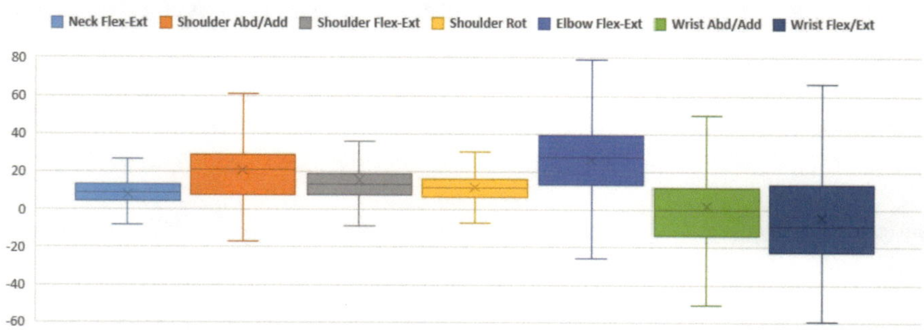

Figure 20.
Results from capture of surgeons' posture performing a simple suture.

5. Effort evaluation

The level of effort involved in the development of work tasks in a particular job is a risk factor for musculoskeletal pathologies. In this sense, different instrumental techniques and electronic measurement systems are used to evaluate the level of effort, such as electromyography (**Figure 21**), which allows to characterize the intensity of muscle intervention of a specific muscle and detect muscle fatigue if it occurs. Force sensors such as force plates allow to measure the reaction force with the environment, and contact pressure sensors allow to measure the pressure that the surgeon experiences when holding and manipulating laparoscopic instruments, which also constitutes a risk factor. In the studies carried out by the BioĚrgon Group, surface electromyography (EMG) has been used as an instrumental technique to analyze the relationship of the position adopted by the surgeons.

5.1 Surface electromyography

Electromyographic data were recorded with the surface electrode and were carried out to establish upper trapezius and middle deltoid intervention as neck-shoulder area stabilizers. Thirteen surgeons (four woman and nine men), with different experience levels, performed a surgery simulation of 60 minutes duration at the Jesús Usón Minimally Invasive Surgery Centre, as mentioned in Section 4. The analysis of the electromyographic data in the frequency domain made it possible to detect median frequency (f_{median}) of the appearance of local muscular fatigue (LMF), which is one of the risk factors that cause discomfort and musculoskeletal disorders. Surgery time was divided into 60 intervals with a duration of 1 minute each. In each interval, an EMG record was made, meaning that a period of 1 minute passed between one record and the next. Results show that LFM appears in 62% of analyzed surgeons in part of the analyzed muscles (**Table 1**).

Therefore, it would be advisable to pay special attention to work-rest guidelines, especially for female surgeons. Taking into account the results of the kinematic analysis, it can be stated that the combination of abduction with the elevation of the arms is associated with a high activity of the deltoid and results in the appearance of muscle fatigue that was detected. The appearance of local muscle fatigue has also been confirmed in another study conducted in collaboration between BioĚrgon Group and CCMIJU, where the same methodology as described above was used. Eight experienced surgeons in laparoscopy and LESS (>100 laparoscopic

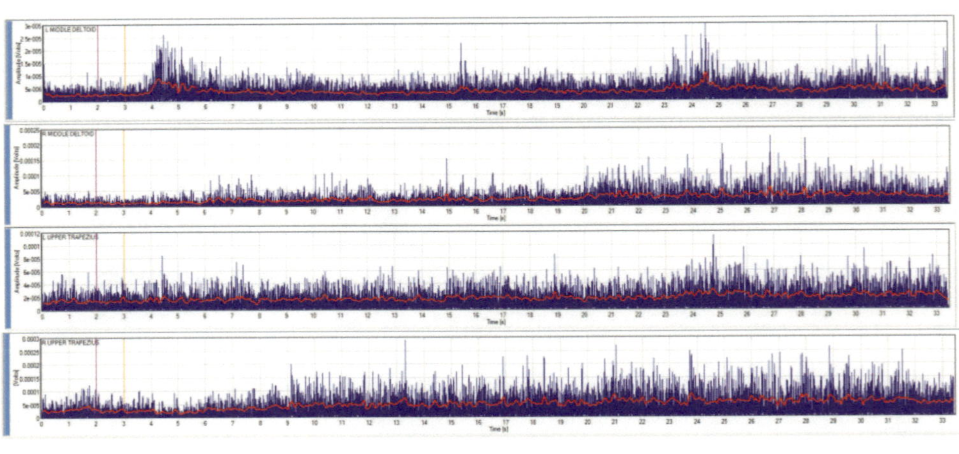

Figure 21.
EMG signal. Blue: rectified signal and red: RMS_{EMG}.

	p-Value	T	r	R^2
01 RT f_{MEAN} 40–60	0.0023**	−4.21	−0.81	66.32%
02 RT f_{MEAN} 20–40	0.0023**	−3.77	−0.72	52.20%
02 RT f_{MEAN} 40–60	0.0085**	−3.19	−0.69	48.00%
02 LT f_{MEAN} 20–40	0.0038**	−3.51	−0.69	48.66%
03 LT f_{MEAN} 0–20	0.0000***	−5.38	−0.79	63.00%
03 LD f_{MEAN} 20–40	0.0025**	−3.54	−0.65	42.46%
04 RD f_{MEAN} 20–40	0.0302*	−2.36	−0.50	24.75%
04 RT f_{MEAN} 40–60	0.0106*	−3.45	−0.79	63.01%
06 LD f_{MEAN} 20–40	0.0000***	−5.95	−0.85	73.13%
07 RD f_{MEAN} 40–60	0.0095**	−3.20	−0.71	50.60%
08 LT f_{MEAN} 20–40	0.005**	−3.49	−0.72	52.65%
08 LD f_{MEAN} 20–40	0.0092**	−3.15	−0.69	47.45%
09 LD f_{MEAN} 20–40	0.0375*	−2.56	−0.69	48.38%
11 TD f_{MEAN} 0–20	0.0358*	−3.63	−0.90	81.50%

*$p \leq 0.05$.
**$p \leq 0.01$.
***$p \leq 0.001$.

Table 1.
Results of LMF observed cases. RT, right trapezius; LT, left trapezius; RD, right deltoid; LD, left deltoid.

procedures and >20 single incision procedures) performed a dissection of the serosa layer of a porcine stomach, attempting to separate the serosa layer from the muscular layers. The single port approach led to significantly greater muscle activity in the paraspinal muscles of the right middle cervical portion and the upper right trapezius than the conventional laparoscopic approach. In both approaches, surgeons showed muscle fatigue in at least one of the analyzed muscles. During dissection using a conventional laparoscopic approach, seven of the surgeons reported muscle fatigue in the upper left trapezius. In the case of the single port approach, seven of the surgeons showed muscle fatigue in the right middle trapezius and they showed increased muscle activity in the paraspinal muscles of the right middle cervical portion and in the right upper trapezius. In both procedures, significant EMG spectral shifts toward lower frequencies were seen in at least one muscle in all surgeons, except for one surgeon during LESS. Significant differences were found for the right upper trapezius and mid-cervical paraspinal muscles ($F[1, 7] > 6.65$ and $p < 0.05$). With the introduction of the instruments with new features and design [35] in the market, comparative studies are carried out with the aim of verifying their functionality and usability. One of the performed studies involved three experienced laparoscopic surgeons carrying out three intracorporeal cutting tasks on a box trainer using a conventional laparoscopic Maryland dissector and a pair of scissors as well as their equivalent r2 DRIVE instruments. Surgeon ergonomics were evaluated through analysis of the surface electromyography of trapezius, deltoid, and paravertebral muscles. Results show that muscle activity of the surgeons was significantly higher for the left deltoid muscle and bilaterally for the muscle trapezius when the novel instruments are used (**Figure 22**).

Finally, twelve laparoscopic partial nephrectomies of the caudal pole in an experimental porcine model were performed by two experienced laparoscopic surgeons, using conventional laparoscopic instruments and laparoscopic instruments with

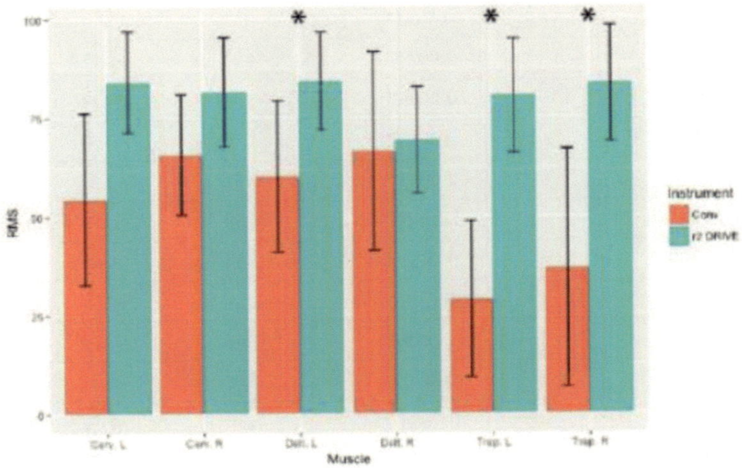

Figure 22.
Muscle activity (RMS_{EMG}) of the paravertebral, deltoid, and trapezius muscles during the use of the conventional and r2 DRIVE laparoscopic instruments.

articulated handle with rings. Results confirmed that although the novel instruments have a new design that incorporates ergonomic criteria, they produced localized muscle fatigue in the left deltoid and bilaterally in the lower trapezius muscles when using the dissector. Even though the surgeons did not notice differences in use and physical workload, the new instruments led to localized muscle fatigue.

5.2 Localized contact pressure

Finally, the last relevant risk factor in the surgical context is **localized contact pressure** (**Figure 23**) that can cause nerve injuries and injuries of the tissue below the skin, especially when it is carried out in a repeated way or when it is maintained for a long time, situations that typically occur during laparoscopic surgery. Sensors and electronic systems are used to record the level and distribution of pressure during the manipulation of laparoscopic instruments (**Figure 23**). This technology allows to evaluate if the pressure levels are harmful for the surgeon and to draw conclusions on the most suitable design of the contact surfaces of the laparoscopic material [36].

Two studies performed in collaboration between CCMIJU and BioÈrgon Group surgeons carried out a urethrovesical anastomosis on a porcine model using a novel handheld robotic laparoscopic instrument and a conventional axial handheld laparoscopic needle holder (two experienced surgeons >100 laparoscopic procedures in the first study and five experienced surgeons in the second one). On the one hand, results show that the pressure exerted by the thumb is notably higher during the use of the robotic instrument. This is due to the interaction with the controls installed on the handle of the instrument. The pressures registered by the index and middle finger as well as the palm of the hand are very similar when using both types of laparoscopic instruments, except for the thumb finger [36]. On the other hand, results showed that the force exerted by the distal phalange of the index finger was significantly higher on the conventional handle as compared to the force exerted on the handle of the robotic instrument. The palm of the hand was the area that received the highest pressure in both instruments, but for longer periods when using the robotic instrument. However, further studies are required to analyze the pressure applied on these laparoscopic instruments by other parts of the hands, such as the intermediate phalanges of the thumb, index, and middle fingers [37].

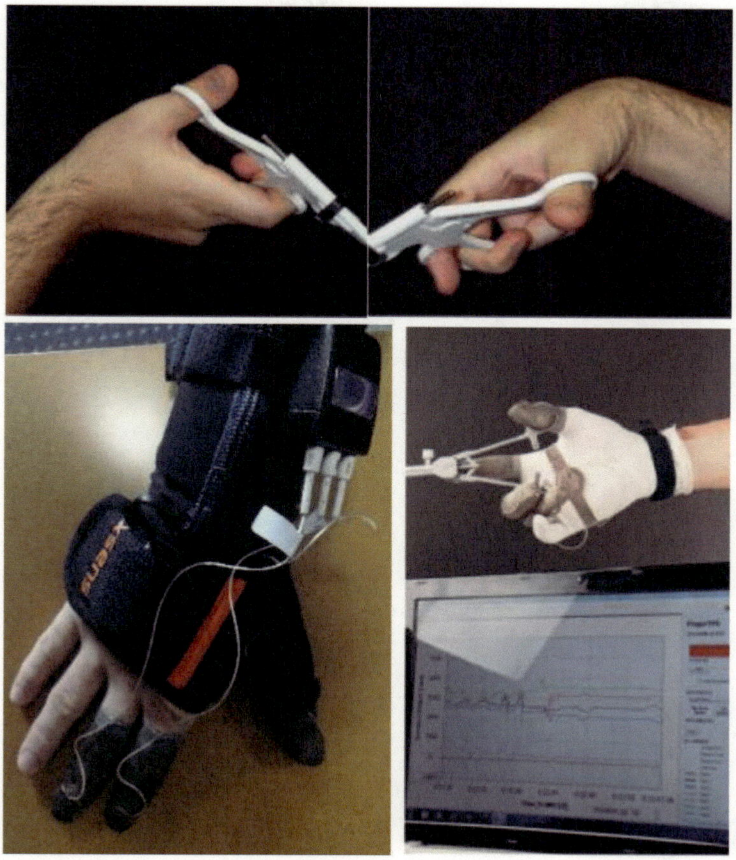

Figure 23.
Contact pressure measurement, generated during the use of laparoscopic instrumental.

6. Conclusion

In this chapter, results of the research work carried out by the collaboration between the BioĚrgon Research Group and the Jesús Usón Minimally Invasive Surgery Centre (CCMIJU) during the last 15 years have been presented. This research was performed based on the methodology of ergonomics, using the instrumental techniques of the Biomechanics of Human Movement to analyze the presence of risk factors of musculoskeletal pathologies in the multiple tasks of laparoscopic surgery and to establish ergonomic criteria that allow to improve the working conditions of surgeons, as well as the design of the laparoscopic material. Results of the research are useful for organizational and ergonomic decision-making, aimed at the introduction of an ergonomic conception of laparoscopic surgery processes for the improvement of occupational health and quality of life of the surgeons. Factors and levels of risk of suffering musculoskeletal injuries in the neck and shoulder associated with posture and muscular activity have been determined, which can be used for the prevention of musculoskeletal pathologies. In addition, the knowledge what was gathered from the real environment of the operating theater can be useful for training of surgeons in laparoscopic surgery on adaptation of the posture during the intervention. Finally, it is relevant to highlight the whole research process conducted for more than a decade, starting from the initial epidemiological study and evolving with the use of biomechanics methodology up to the analysis of neuromuscular control strategies using the uncontrolled manifold hypothesis model.

Acknowledgements

This work was granted by the Government of Extremadura, Spain (Grant Ref. GR18191); and project "Centro de Tecnificación del Deporte Paralímpico – DEPATECH 2014-2015".

Author details

Kostas Gianikellis[1], Andreas Skiadopoulos[2], Rafael Gutiérrez Horrillo[1], Miguel Rodal[1*], Juan Alberto Sánchez-Margallo[3] and Francisco M. Sánchez-Margallo[3]

1 BioẼrgon Research Group, Biomechanics of Human Movement and Ergonomics Lab, University of Extremadura, Cáceres, Spain

2 Department of Biomechanics and Center for Research in Human Movement Variability, University of Nebraska Omaha, Omaha, NE, USA

3 Jesús Usón Minimally Invasive Surgery Centre, Cáceres, Spain

*Address all correspondence to: mrodal@unex.es

References

[1] Gianikellis K. El Diseño Ergonómico en el Mueble. Cáceres: Cámara de Comercio de Cáceres; 2001

[2] Dankelman J, Grimbergen CA, Stassen HG. Observation and Manipulation in Laparoscopic Surgery. Engineering for Patient Safety: CRC Press; 2004. pp. 66-111

[3] Berquer R, Smith WD, Davis S. An ergonomic study of the optimum operating table height for laparoscopic surgery. Surgical Endoscopy. 2002;**16**(3):416-421

[4] Zehetner J, Kaltenbacher A, Wayand W, Shamiyeh A. Screen height as an ergonomic factor in laparoscopic surgery. Surgical Endoscopy. 2006;**20**(1):139-141

[5] Berguer R, Forkey DL, Smith WD. The effect of laparoscopic instrument working angle on surgeons' upper extremity workload. Surgical Endoscopy. 2001;**15**(9):1027-1029

[6] Berguer R, Forkey DL, Smith WD. Ergonomic problems associated with laparoscopic surgery. Surgical Endoscopy. 1999;**13**(5):466-468

[7] Berguer R, Remler M, Beckley D. Laparoscopic instruments cause increased forearm fatigue: A subjective and objective comparison of open and laparoscopic techniques. Minimally Invasive Therapy & Allied Technologies. 1997;**6**(1):36-40

[8] Horgan LF, Oriordan DC, Doctor N. Neuropraxia following laparoscopic procedures: An occupational injury. Minimally Invasive Therapy & Allied Technologies. 1997;**6**(1):33-35

[9] Kano N, Yamakawa T, Kasugai H. Laparoscopic surgeon's thumb. Archives of Surgery. 1993;**128**(10):1172

[10] Sanchez-Margallo FM, Gianikellis K, Skiadopoulos A, Hermoso-deMendoza J, Sanchez-Margallo JA. Localized muscle fatigue in laparoendoscopic single site surgery and conventional laparoscopic. In: 23rd International Congress of the European Association for Endoscopic Surgery (EAES). 2016. Available from: https://link.springer.com/content/pdf/10.1007/s00464-016-4766-4.pdf2016

[11] Sánchez-Margallo FM, Sánchez-Margallo JA, Gutiérrez R, Rodal M, Brun MV, Gianikellis K. Analysis of a novel handheld robotic needle holder: Surgical skills and ergonomics. In: MISWeek 2018-SLS Annual Meeting. 2018

[12] Sánchez-Margallo JA, Sánchez-Margallo FM, Gutiérrez R, Rodal M, Veloso-Brun M, Gianikellis K. Surgical performance and muscle fatigue using a novel articulated laparoscopic instrument handle with rings: Study in a porcine model. In: 53rd Congress of the European Society for Surgical Research (ESSR). 2018. Available from: https://www.essr2018.com/abstracts2018

[13] Boer Den K, Gouma D, Grimbergen C, Dankelman J. Evaluation of the surgical process. In: Lawrence Erlbaum Associates I, editor. Engineering for Patient Safety: Issues in Minimally Invasive Procedures. Mahwah, New Jersey: CRC Press; 2004. pp. 20-43

[14] Patkin M, Isabel L. Ergonomics, engineering and surgery of endosurgical dissection. Journal of the Royal College of Surgeons of Edinburgh. 1995;**40**(2):120-132

[15] OSHA. Work-Related Neck and Upper Limb Musculoskeletal Disorders: European Agency for Safety and Health at Work; 1999

[16] Rodigari A, Bejor M, Carlisi E, Lisi C, Tinelli C, Toffola E. Identification of

risk factors for fatigue and pain when performing surgical interventions. Giornale Italiano di Medicina del Lavoro ed Ergonomia. 2012;**34**(4):432-437

[17] Kuorinka I, Jonsson B, Kilbom A, Vinterberg H, Biering-Sørensen F, Andersson G, et al. Standardised Nordic questionnaires for the analysis of musculoskeletal symptoms. Applied Ergonomics. 1987;**18**(3):233-237

[18] Dickinson CE, Campion K, Foster AF, Newman SJ, Orourke AMT, Thomas PG. Questionnaire development—An examination of the nordic musculoskeletal questionnaire. Applied Ergonomics. 1992;**23**(3):197-201

[19] Cohen A, Gjessing C, Fine LA. Primer Based on Workplace Evaluations of Musculoskeletal Disorders. Vol. 97-117. US Department of Health and Human Services, National Institute for Occupational Safety and Health, DHHS (NIOSH) Publication; 1997. pp. 16-30

[20] Manukyan GA, Waseda M, Inaki N, Bermudez JRT, Gacek IA, Rudinski A, et al. Ergonomics with the use of curved versus straight laparoscopic graspers during rectosigmoid resection: Results of a multiprofile comparative study. Surgical Endoscopy. 2007;**21**(7):1079-1089

[21] Gianikellis K, Fernández J, Gazo A, Skiadopoulos A, Pantrigo JJ. Diseño y Desarrollo del Paquete informático "Biomsoft" 2.0 y Su aplicación al análisis de la Marcha Humana Normal y patológica. XXXIII Congreso de la Sociedad ibérica de biomecánica y Biomateriales. 2010

[22] Eronomics Principles to Workspace Desing; 2004

[23] Karhu O, Kansi P, Kuorinka I. Correcting working postures in industry—practical method for analysis. Applied Ergonomics. 1977;**8**(4):199-201

[24] Wu G, van der Helm FCT, Veeger HEJ, Makhsous M, Van Roy P, Anglin C, et al. ISB recommendation on definitions of joint coordinate systems of various joints for the reporting of human joint motion—Part II: Shoulder, elbow, wrist and hand. Journal of Biomechanics. 2005;**38**(5):981-992

[25] Gianikellis K. Desarrollo de una metodología Para análisis biomecánico en los deportes de precisión. Aplicación en el tiro olímpico; 1996

[26] Grood ES, Suntay WJ. A joint coordinate system for the clinical description of three-dimensional motions: Application to the knee. Journal of Biomechanical Engineering. 1983;**105**(2):136-144

[27] Marras WS. Occupational biomechanics. In: The Occupational Ergonomics Handbook. Florida, USA: CRC Press LLC; 1999. pp. 167-204

[28] Skiadopoulos A, Espino-Palma C, Gianikellis K. Upper Extremity 3d Kinematics and Musculoskeletal Effort in Laparoscopy. ESB; 2013. Available from: http://esbiomech.org/papers/ESB_congress_2013/oral/S61.3-561.pdf2013

[29] Nguyen NT, Ho HS, Smith WD, Philipps C, Lewis C, De Vera RM, et al. An ergonomic evaluation of surgeons' axial skeletal and upper extremity movements during laparoscopic and open surgery. American Journal of Surgery. 2001;**182**(6):720-724

[30] Vereczkei A, Feussner H, Negele T, Fritzsche F, Seitz T, Bubb H, et al. Ergonomic assessment of the static stress confronted by surgeons during laparoscopic cholecystectomy. Surgical Endoscopy. 2004;**18**(7):1118-1122

[31] Nisky I, Hsieh MH, Okamura AM. A framework for analysis of surgeon arm posture variability in robot-assisted surgery. In: IEEE International

Conference on Robotics and Automation (ICRA). New York: IEEE; 2013. pp. 245-251

[32] Gianikellis K, Skiadopoulos A, Palma CE, Sanchez-Margallo FM, Carrasco JBP, Sanchez-Margallo JA, et al. Method to assess upper-body postural variability in laparoscopic surgery. In: 2014 5th IEEE RAS & EMBS International Conference on Biomedical Robotics and Biomechatronics. Proceedings of the IEEE RAS-EMBS International Conference on Biomedical Robotics and Biomechatronics. New York: IEEE; 2014. pp. 76-81

[33] Gianikellis K, Sanchez-Margallo FM, Skiadopoulos A, Sanchez-Margallo JA, Aranda JHD. Head stabilization during minimal invasive surgery tasks: An uncontrolled manifold analysis. In: Ahram T, Karwowski W, Schmorrow D, editors. 6th International Conference on Applied Human Factors and Ergonomics. Procedia Manufacturing 3. Amsterdam: Elsevier Science B.V; 2015. pp. 1434-1441

[34] Sánchez-Margallo JA, Sánchez-Margallo FM, Gianikellis K, Skiadopoulos A, Hermoso J. 3D Kinematics of Surgeons' Upper-Arm Rotation in Laparoscopy. SMIT; 2016. Available from: http://www.smit2016.com/iSMIT-AbstractsBook.pdf2016

[35] Bekku A, Kim J, Nakajima Y, Yonenobu K. A body-mounted surgical assistance robot for minimally invasive spinal puncture surgery. In: 2014 5th IEEE RAS & EMBS International Conference on Biomedical Robotics and Biomechatronics. Proceedings of the IEEE RAS-EMBS International Conference on Biomedical Robotics and Biomechatronics. New York: IEEE; 2014. pp. 19-23

[36] Sanchez-Margallo JA, Sanchez-Margallo FM, Skiadopoulos A, Lango T, Gianikellis K, editors. Analysis of the Pressure Exerted by the Surgeon's Hand and Fingers Using a Novel Robotic Laparoscopic Instrument during Urethrovesical Anastomosis. Society of American Gastrointestinal and Endoscopic Surgeons (SAGES); 2016. Available from: https://www.sages.org/meetings/annual-meeting/abstracts-archive/analysis-of-the-pressure-exerted-by-the-surgeons-hand-and-fingers-using-a-novel-robotic-laparoscopic-instrument-during-urethrovesical-anastomosis/2016

[37] Sánchez-Margallo JA, Sánchez-Margallo FM, Gianikellis K, Skiadopoulos A, Hermoso J, Lango T, editors. Surgical performance and ergonomics of the surgeon's hand using a robotic handheld needle holder. In: 28th Conference of the International Society for Medical Innovation and Technology; Delft, The Netherlands. 2016. Available from: http://www.smit2016.com/iSMIT-AbstractsBook.pdf

Section 2

Gastrointestinal Surgery

Chapter 3

Endoluminal Techniques to Treat Obesity

Suzanne Pruijssers, Ernst van Heurn and Nicole Bouvy

Abstract

The prevalence of overweight and obesity increased dramatically during the past decades and now affects approximately 30% of people worldwide. Bariatric surgery has proven to be the most effective treatment modality for obesity in the long term. However, current surgical procedures are accompanied by a substantial risk of complications. Several endoluminal techniques have been developed to achieve weight loss in obese patients and claim to be as effective as surgery but safer. This chapter evaluates the efficacy and safety of innovative endoluminal techniques that are already available in clinical practice or in advanced stages of development. This chapter outlines their potential mechanism of action and their safety and efficacy in clinical practice, by reviewing the current literature.

Keywords: endoscopic, endoluminal, laparoscopic, obesity, bariatric

1. Introduction

Overweight and obesity have reached epidemic proportions. The World Health Organization (WHO) estimates that approximately 2.5 billion adults are overweight, and at least 700 million are obese [1]. Overweight and obesity are linked to more deaths worldwide than underweight. As the number of people with obesity rises, the prevalence of obesity-related comorbidities, such as diabetes, hypertension, hyperlipidemia, obstructive sleep apnea, and fatty-liver disease is rising as well. Numerous strategies have been employed in the treatment of obesity; however, most people do not reach or sustain such significant weight loss with lifestyle intervention, composed of diet, exercise, and behavior modification, alone. Bariatric surgery has emerged as the most effective treatment for obesity in the long term and is associated with a significant decrease in obesity-associated comorbidities [2, 3]. However, current bariatric surgical procedures are accompanied by a substantial risk of complications. These potentially serious complications during and following the invasive and irreversible surgical procedures are incontrovertible. In addition, only a small proportion of obese patients actually undergo bariatric surgery. With this in mind, there exists a critical gap in the treatment of obesity for those not qualifying for bariatric surgery or those who do not wish to pursue bariatric surgery because of a multitude of reasons such as the associated risks, morbidity, and costs. Thus, there is a strong need for new and less invasive, safer and preferably reversible alternatives to bariatric surgical procedures. Therefore, new techniques to achieve weight loss in obese patients who claim to be as effective as surgery but safer have been developed. In addition, these therapies may be beneficial earlier on in the onset of obesity. In this chapter, we aim to present the current state of field regarding investigational procedures in the treatment of obesity that are already available in clinical practice or in advanced stages of development. This chapter outlines their potential mechanism of action and their safety and efficacy in clinical practice, by reviewing the current literature.

2. Malabsorptive procedures

2.1 Gastrointestinal bypass liners

With the success of the Roux-Y Gastric Bypass (RYGB), attempts have been made to develop nonsurgical endoscopic procedures which mimic the attributes of the RYGB. Several companies have come up with gastrointestinal bypass liners which are removable, replaceable, and do not require gastric stapling or permanent changes to the patient's anatomy.

2.1.1 The EndoBarrier

A promising alternative to bariatric surgery is the EndoBarrier (**Figure 1**) (GI Dynamics Inc., Lexington Massachusetts, USA). This device is an endoluminal duodenal bypass liner (DJBL), which mimics the malabsorptive features of the RYGB.

2.1.1.1 Technique

The EndoBarrier consists of a single use endoscopic system including a liner, delivery system, and retrieval system. The liner, a Teflon covered sleeve that is impermeable to nutrients, extends 65 cm into the small bowel and can remain in situ for up to 3–12 months. Under general anesthesia, a capsule containing the liner and its anchor will be placed at the duodenal bulb with fluoroscopic guidance. The device has anchors with barbs of nitinol located at its proximal end, which functions as a self-expandable stent. This allows fixation to the duodenal bulb distal to the pylorus, but proximal to the ampulla of Vater. In this way, the liner is anchored proximally, whereas the distal part extends into the jejunum due to peristalsis of the intestine. The liner is open at both sides, to ensure the passage of chyme from the stomach while bypassing the duodenum. Along the outside of the liner, pancreatic juices and bile will enter from the ampulla of Vater, thereby avoiding contact with gastric contents until these exit the sleeve in the jejunum. In this way, it mimics the malabsorptive effects of the RYGB, without the permanent alterations of the intestinal anatomy and its complications. The device is licensed for 1 year, after which it should be removed. In order to remove the liner, a custom drawstring of the device can be grasped with an endoscope, to which the device will collapse and subsequently can be gently removed from the gastrointestinal tract.

2.1.1.2 Efficacy and safety profile

To date, there have been multiple observational studies and five randomized controlled trials assessing the efficacy of the EndoBarrier [4]. The first post marketing nonrandomized trial was conducted in the United Kingdom, in which 45 obese patients with a mean BMI of 39.9 kg/m^2 were recruited [5]. The study comprised a 12-month period with the EndoBarrier inserted and a 6-month follow-up period after it had been explanted. Average implantation time was 27 min and no procedure-related complications occurred. A total of 31/45 patients completed the full 12 month-period, whereas 14 patients had a premature removal of the device. In two patients, this was due to a device-related adverse event, namely melena and device migration causing abdominal pain. In the remaining 31 patients, a mean reduction in BMI of 4.9 kg/m^2 was observed at 12 months. In addition, this reduction in weight was maintained 6 months after the removal of the device. In another study, 41 patients with a mean BMI of 49 kg/m^2 were randomized between the EndoBarrier and a low calorie diet [6]. After 12 weeks, the mean excess weight loss (EWL) in the device group versus the control group was 19 versus 6.9%, respectively. In one large multicenter trial carried out in the Netherlands, 73 patients were randomized to either EndoBarrier implantation in combination with dietary intervention or dietary intervention alone [7]. Thirty-five subjects with a baseline BMI of 35 kg/m^2 received the EndoBarrier for a period of 6 months. After 6 months, just before the device removal, the EndoBarrier group had lost 32.0% [22.0–46.7%] of their excess weight versus 16.4% [4.1–34.6%] in the control group ($p < 0.05$). In addition, the EndoBarrier-group demonstrated the impact on diabetic control, with improvements in HbA1c of 1.3% compared to 0.3% in the control group. Only one early device removal was reported due to the blockage of the Endobarrier with food. A recent systematic review and meta-analysis assessing the effect of the EndoBarrier on weight loss and glycemic control in obese patients with type 2 diabetes mellitus concluded that the EndoBarrier induces significant weight loss and improves glycemic control in this population [8]. With regard to safety, the most frequently reported side effect of the EndoBarrier is abdominal pain and nausea, which commonly resolves after the body is used to having the device in situ. More serious complications that have been reported are gastrointestinal bleeding, device migration, and the formation of hepatic abscesses. However, the first international data from the EndoBarrier worldwide registry suggest that the likely benefits of the EndoBarrier far outweigh the risks. The registry, including 403 Endobarrier patients, reported 4 cases of hepatic abscesses, 15 cases of gastrointestinal bleeding, and 8 cases of device migration [9]. In conclusion, the EndoBarrier has shown to be a promising and feasible technique that is able to account for significant weight loss in obese patients and moreover improves glycemic control in those with T2DM. However, while the liner is currently licensed for only 1 year, a vast majority of the patients risk to lose the beneficial effects of the device after removal and subsequently will regain weight. In the study of Forner et al., 72% of the patients regained their weight 6 months postremoval of the EndoBarrier [10]. Future research should be focused on reimplantation strategies or a device that could

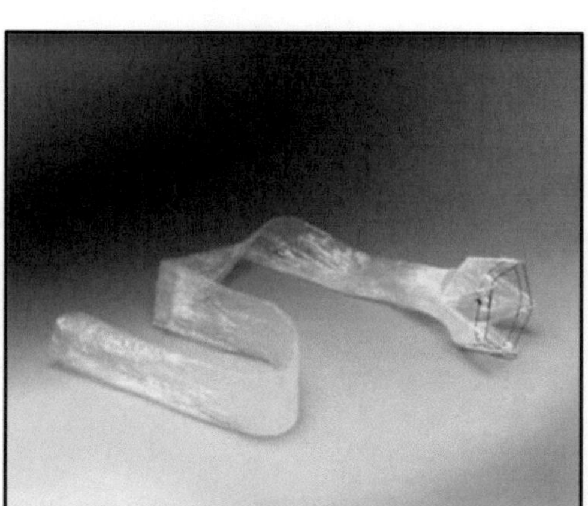

Figure 1.
The EndoBarrier.

remain in situ for longer, thereby providing a more permanent solution. A recent study already demonstrated implantation of a new prototype for up to 3 years in two obese subjects with T2DM, but high frequency and severity of AE's still preclude the use of the device for a period longer than 1 year [11]. Efforts are made to kick start further development to combat these issues.

2.1.2 ValenTx

Another novel endoluminal gastro duodenal-jejunal bypass liner which has been introduced is the ValenTx (**Figure 2**) (ValenTx, Inc. Carpinteria, CA, USA) [12]. It is designed to reproduce the restrictive and malabsorptive features of the RYGB, by creating a gastric, duodenal, and biliopancreatic bypass. This gastro duodenal-jejunal bypass liner is an implantation device which is delivered endoscopically, but other than the EndoBarrier, requires laparoscopic assistance.

2.1.2.1 Technique

The procedure starts with an overtube placed through the pylorus at the level of the duodenal bulb. The liner, a 120-cm long fluoropolymer, is then delivered through this overtube via a delivery catheter up till the first portion of the duodenum. The liner, which has a polyester cuff attached to its proximal end, is deployed using computer-regulated pressure and flow monitoring under fluoroscopic guidance to ensure deployment of the liner into the proximal jejunum. Hereafter, the delivery catheter will be removed, and the overtube will be replaced for a shorter one leading up to the proximal cuff attachment. After this step, the laparoscopic part of the procedure will take place. After the placement of one 12-mm and three 5-mm trocars together with a Nathanson liver retractor, the gastroesophageal (GE) junction is dissected circumferentially at the level of the diaphragmatic hiatus. With an endoscope, the polyester cuff will then be positioned at the level of the Z-line of the GE junction and anchored with full-thickness sutures deployed in a circumferential manner. Full-thickness suture placement is secured under laparoscopic visualization. After cuff attachment, the final step in the procedure is approximation of the left and right diaphragmatic crura through laparoscopically placed sutures to prevent iatrogenic hiatal hernia. In order to remove the device, one has to circumferentially detach the cuff by endoscopic ligation of the eight anchoring sutures. The cuff can then be gently mobilized with an endoscopic grasper and subsequently be removed via the esophagus together with the attached sleeve.

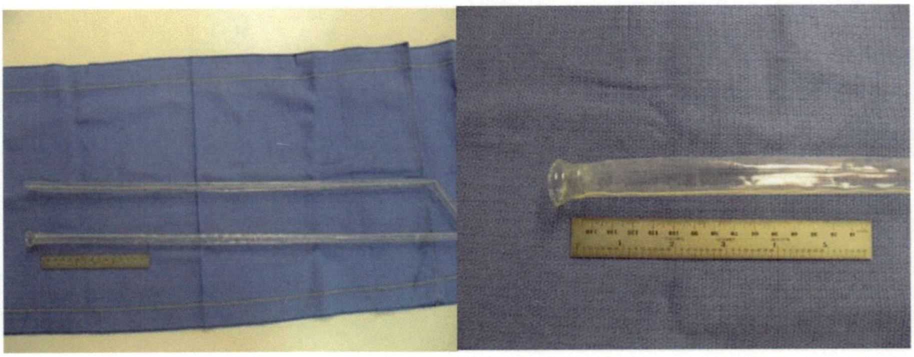

Figure 2.
The ValenTx gastro duodenal-jejunal bypass liner ([12], with permission).

2.1.2.2 Efficacy and safety profile

The first human experience with the ValenTx was gained during a single-center prospective trial among 24 morbidly obese individuals who met the National Institutes of Health (NIH) criteria for bariatric surgery [12]. In 22 patients, with a mean preoperative BMI of 42 kg/m^2, the liner was successfully implanted. One patient got excluded because of noncompliance with the preoperative liquid diet, and another patient suffered from significant inflammation at the GE junction to which the investigators decided to halt the procedure. A total of 5 out of the 22 implanted patients underwent the removal of the liner before the 12-week scheduled explantation, because of dysphagia presumably due to a too high placement of the cuff. This complaint completely resolved after explantation of the liner. After 12 weeks, the average % EWL in the successfully implanted patients was 39.7% (27–64%), which corresponded with an average total weight loss of 16.8 kg (8.6–30.8 kg). Moreover, the device demonstrated effective glycemic control during the trial. Except for the patients requiring premature explantation, no other adverse events took place. Therefore, the same research group designed a consecutive 1-year trial in which 13 patients with a mean BMI of 42 kg/m^2 were enrolled [13]. In 10 patients, the device was successfully implanted and left in situ for 12 months. All 10 patients completed the 1-year follow-up without major complications resulting in a mean % EWL of 54% after 1-year and significant improvement of all comorbidities. Partial cuff detachment was observed in four patients during follow-up endoscopy, which indicates that the redesign of the anchoring mechanism is needed before further research can be done. While showing to be safe and able to achieve significant weight loss, further research is focused on a purely endoscopic deployment of this device. Unfortunately, further development and research on this device is currently hampered due to investment problems.

3. Restrictive procedures

Restrictive procedures limit food intake, creating a small gastric reservoir with a narrow outlet to delay gastric emptying, thereby stimulating an earlier sense of satiety with reduction of caloric intake.

3.1 Gastric remodeling techniques

3.1.1 TOGA system

Transoral gastroplasty (TOGA) with the use of the TOGA system (Satiety Inc., Palo Alto, CA) creates a vertical gastroplasty along the lesser curvature of the stomach performed through a transoral endoscopy [14]. The created gastric pouch limits the amount of food or liquids that the patient can eat, with an accompanying feeling of early satiety.

3.1.1.1 Technique

The TOGA is an incision free procedure performed under general anesthesia creating a restrictive pouch in the stomach using a set of flexible staplers which are introduced endoscopically. Using suction, tissue from both the anterior and posterior wall of the stomach is positioned together into two vacuum pods inside the device. Hereafter, 3 rows of 11 titanium staples create a serosa to serosa transmural suture, connecting the anterior and posterior gastric walls from the angle of His to the lesser curvature. This step is repeated until one has created a sleeve of the desired length. The sleeve outlet is then narrowed using the TOGA restrictor.

3.1.1.2 Efficacy and safety profile

The first human study assessing the safety and efficacy of the TOGA system took place in 2008, in which 21 morbidly obese individuals with a mean BMI of 43.4 kg/m^2 were enrolled [15]. After 6 months, patients had an average EWL of 24.4%. No serious adverse events (SAE) were reported. However, at 6 month follow-up endoscopy, gaps in the staple line were observed in 13 out of 21 patients. After technical improvements of the device, a second human pilot study enrolled 11 patients who met criteria for bariatric surgery [14]. Average BMI decreased significantly from 41.6 kg/m^2 before treatment to 33.1 kg/m^2 at 6 month follow-up. The same results were seen in a multicenter trial with 1-year outcome, which involved 67 patients with a mean BMI of 41.5 kg/m^2, which dropped to 33.1 kg/m^2 at 6 months after the TOGA procedure [16]. A small case study evaluating the effect of TOGA on insulin sensitivity and secretion even demonstrated an amelioration of insulin sensitivity with subsequent reduction of the insulin secretion [17]. Compared to the more effective laparoscopic gastric bypass and biliopancreatic diversion, the TOGA system reached a good therapeutic outcome in terms of weight loss and showed no complications [18]. Based on the evidence available, TOGA has showed to be a feasible and effective procedure to treat obesity with a promising potential for the future. However, a multicenter randomized FDA trial was terminated secondary to lack of efficacy, whereafter the company dissolved, and future applications remain uncertain.

3.1.2 Endoscopic sleeve gastroplasty (ESG)

Another system to create a restrictive sleeve is the Overstitch system (Apollo Endosurgery, Austin, Texas, USA). Contrary to the TOGA system, it applies full-thickness running sutures alongside the greater curvature of the stomach. This results in a reduction of the functional capacity of the stomach by up to 70%, a size comparable to the reduction of the gastric lumen in laparoscopic sleeve gastrectomy (LSG) [19]. This device is currently commercially available in the United States.

3.1.2.1 Technique

The Overstitch system (**Figure 3**) consists of a double-channel endoscope equipped with a mounted suturing platform. To ensure full-thickness suture placement, a tissue grasper device is used to mobilize and capture the desired location of the suture at the gastric wall, whereafter the tissue is retracted into the suturing arm of the device [20]. As the evolution of the ESG evolved over time, different

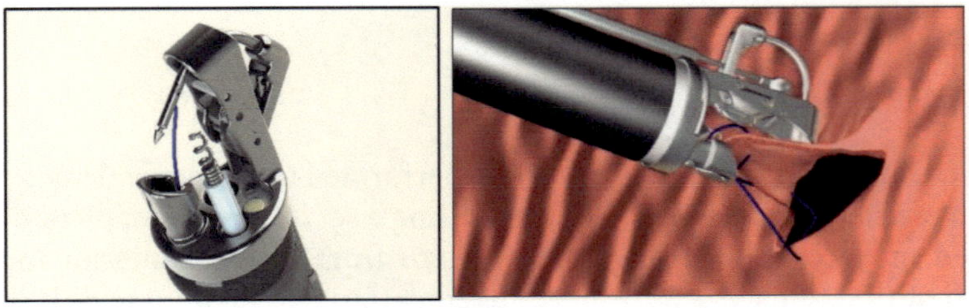

Figure 3.
The Overstitch system and full-thickness suture placement (from ApolloEndosurgery®, with permission).

techniques of suture placement have been tried, and therefore vary between studies [21]. A recent study showed good effect of a modified running suture following a Z-pattern, to provide a homogenous distribution of the disruptive force on the suture among all stitch points [22].

3.1.2.2 Efficacy and safety profile

After the Mayo Clinic first demonstrated the clinical safety and feasibility of this technique in early 2013, multiple studies have confirmed the safety and efficacy of this procedure. A multicenter study among 3 centers, including 248 subjects with a baseline BMI of 37.8 ± 5.6 kg/m^2, showed a total body weight loss (TBWL) of 15.2% [95%CI 14.2–16.3] and 18.6% [15.7–21.5], at, respectively, 6 and 24 month follow-up [23]. Five (2%) serious adverse events occurred: two patients presented with peri-gastric inflammatory fluid collection which resolved with percutaneous drainage and antibiotics, one patient presented with self-limiting hemorrhage due to marginal splenic laceration, one patient with a pulmonary embolism 72 h postoperative, and one patient required placement of a chest tube to treat concomitant pneumoperitoneum and pneumothorax caused during the procedure. All patients recovered without the need of surgical intervention. A recent retrospective analysis among 112 obese patients (baseline BMI 37.9 ± 6.7 kg/m^2) who underwent ESG using the Overstitch device reported comparable and consistent findings of approximately 15% TBWL and 50% EWL at 6 month post-ESG [24]. In the prospective study of Sharaiha et al., ESG accounted for a reduction in markers of hypertension, diabetes, and hypertriglyceridemia in addition to sustained total body weight loss after a period of 24 months [25]. ESG appears to be safe and effective in obese patients, but future randomized research is needed before incorporation into clinical practice can take place.

3.1.3 Primary obesity surgery endoluminal (POSE)

The POSE procedure is an approach in which a reduction of the gastric fundus is created, using a peroral incisionless operating platform (USGI Medical. San Clemente, CA, USA) [26]. During this procedure, transmural plications are placed at eight to nine locations in the gastric fundus with an additional three plications in de distal part of the stomach. The notion behind this is to mechanically and physically restrict the surface to which ingested food comes in contact with the stomach. Moreover, it is assumed that the plications in the gastric fundus limit the capacity to accommodate food, and therefore, activation of gastric stretch receptors in response to food is more rapidly induced.

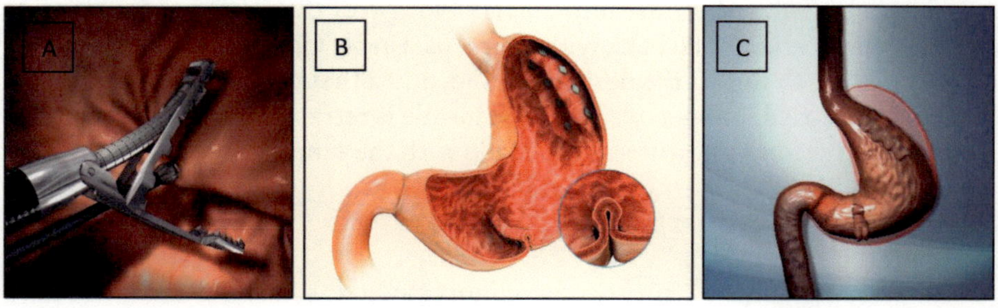

Figure 4.
The g-Prox EZ® Endoscopic Grasper (A), transmural plications at the gastric fundus and distal part of the stomach (B), and stomach after POSE procedure (C) (from USGI Medical®, with permission).

3.1.3.1 Technique

In order to create full-thickness serosa-to-serosa plications, a special overtube-style platform, the Transport Endoscopic Access Device (USGI medical) is used at the operative site [26]. It has four working channels through which an endoscope and three additional instruments can be introduced. The g-Prox EZ® Endoscopic Grasper, a flexible shaft with a gripper at the tip to mobilize and capture target tissue (**Figure 4A**); the g-Lix™ Tissue Grasper, a flexible probe which is designed to assist the g-Prox in capturing the desired tissue; and the g-Cath EZ™ Suture Anchor Delivery Catheter which is equipped with a needle at its distal tip, and facilitates the creating of plications by penetrating the mobilized tissue with a pair of pre-loaded suture anchors. This ensures anchoring of the fold until there is serosal fusion.

3.1.3.2 Efficacy and safety profile

Current literature on the efficacy and safety of this device consists of two-open label prospective single-arm trials and two randomized controlled trials [26–29]. In a multicenter randomized controlled trial in the United States, 221 patients received the POSE procedure combined with low-intensity lifestyle interventions for a period of 12 months [29]. They achieved a TBWL of 4.95 ± 7.04%, in comparison to 1.38 ± 5.58% in the control group, consisting of 111 patients who received low-intensity lifestyle intervention alone. Reported SAE were 4.7% (1.9% vomiting, 1.6% nausea, and 0.4% pain), which often occurred within the first week post-procedure and required extended hospital stay. In addition, 0.4% extra gastric bleeding and 0.4% liver abscess occurred which required, respectively, open surgery and percutaneous drainage [29, 30]. In another multicenter randomized controlled trial, POSE-treated subjects showed 30% TBWL after 12 months compared to 5.9% in the control group [28]. Furthermore, the POSE procedure has demonstrated to result in a significant improvement in satiation [31]. In conclusion, the POSE procedure is a promising option for the bariatric patient, but still requires further development.

3.1.4 Endomina system

The Endomina system (EndoTool SA [SST], Gosselies, Belgium) reduces gastric volume by creating an endoscopic gastroplasty alongside the greater curvature of the stomach [32].

3.1.4.1 Technique

By using an over-the-scope triangulation platform attached to an endoscope, anterior-to-posterior greater curvature plications are applied. While introducing a 5F needle preloaded with suture into the flexible arm of the platform, the stomach wall is mobilized and pulled back with a forceps. Under visual control, the needle pierces the stomach wall at the designated site, and a first tag, attached to the suture and a pre-tied knot, is released. The needle is retracted, the first plicature is released, and a second plicature can be made with the same action.

3.1.4.2 Efficacy and safety profile

A single-center, phase 1, prospective cohort study was initiated in May 2015, which demonstrated 11% TWBL after 6 months. No major adverse event was observed in the 10 patients who underwent the procedure [32]. In a multicenter prospective trial with 1-year follow-up, EWL and TBWL at 1 year were 29%

(SD 28) and 7.4% (SD 7), respectively, for the whole cohort (45 patients). At follow-up gastroscopy, 88% of sutures were still in place (30 patients). No SAE were observed [33]. A randomized controlled trial comparing the Endomina combined with diet to diet alone is currently underway.

3.1.5 Articular circular stapling device (ACE)

The articular circular stapling device (**Figure 5**) (BaroSense, Redwood City, CA; Boston Scientific Corp., Marlbourough, MA) is an investigational device which applies full-thickness transmural plications of the stomach wall aided by vacuum and stapling.

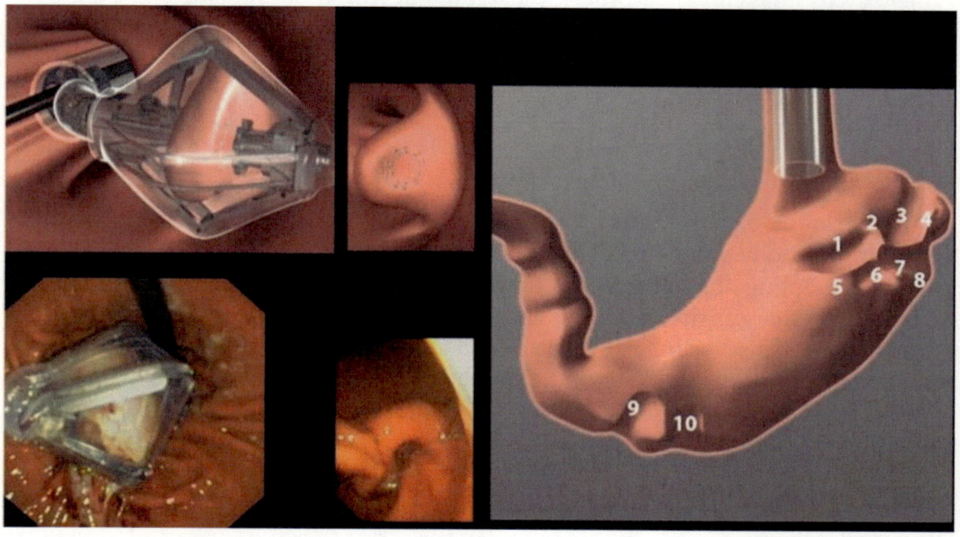

Figure 5.
The ACE stapler: after the tissue is acquired by vacuum, plications are made with a circular staple ring in 10 locations in the stomach (from [34], with permission).

3.1.5.1 Technique

With an outer diameter of 16 mm, the device has a built-in channel for a 5-mm endoscope. The stapler head, located at the distal part of the device, is able to rotate 360° and orientate into complete flexion or retroflexion. When introduced into the stomach, it is able to create a vacuum inside its silicone cover, to capture the desired amount of stomach tissue. After ensuring an adequate amount, the acquired piece of stomach tissue will be compressed by a 10-mm plastic ring with eight titanium staples, thereby creating a large, full-thickness transmural plication. After pre-loading the system with a new staple cartridge, creation of new plications can be continued in the same fashion. After a maximum of eight plications in the fundus together with an additional two in the antrum of the stomach, reduction of stomach volume alongside the greater curvature is completed. The two extra plications in the antrum of the stomach are believed to delay gastric emptying.

3.1.5.2 Efficacy and safety profile

This first reported human phase 1 study enrolled 17 patients with a median BMI of 40.2 kg/m^2 who underwent the ACE procedure [34]. Adverse events involved gastric pain (n = 7), sore throat (n = 4), diarrhea (n = 4), nausea (n = 3), and constipation (n = 4), but resolved with conservative treatment within 15 days after surgery. No SAE occurred. Patients demonstrated a median % EWL of 34.9% (IQR 17.8–46.6) in the first year. This phase 1 study showed that the ACE stapler is safe and effective in humans. The study was funded by Barosense until sufficient funds could no longer been raised and further research was discontinued. However, randomized controlled trials and long-term follow up are needed to determine its place in the treatment of obesity. With acquisition by Boston Scientific Group, follow-up research on the ACE procedure may be on the horizon in the near future.

3.1.6 The incisionless magnetic anastomosis system

The incisionless magnetic anastomosis system (IMA) manufactured by GI Windows (Boston, MA) is a compression anastomosis technology used to create a dual-path enteral bypass in the small bowel with the use of octagon shaped self-assembling magnets.

3.1.6.1 Technique

Under fluoroscopic guidance, self-assembling magnets are delivered in the proximal jejunum and ileum by simultaneous upper and lower endoscopy. After deployment and coupling due to the magnetic field, the tissue in between will be pressed against each other causing necrosis. The necrotized tissue induces remodeling of the surrounding tissue, leading to the formation of a jejunal-ileal anastomosis. After the anastomosis has been established, the coupled magnets will be expelled by the feces.

3.1.6.2 Efficacy and safety profile

Ten patients with a mean BMI of 41 kg/m^2 underwent the procedure in the first human pilot study [35, 36]. In this pilot, laparoscopy assistance was used to ensure adequate magnet coupling and verify limb lengths. The anastomosis was formed in approximately 1 week, and magnets were expelled without pain or obstruction. All anastomoses were patent at 2- and 6-month follow-up endoscopy. After 6 months, subject demonstrated a TBWL of 10.6%. After 1 year, EWL was 40.2%, and all anastomosis remained patent. No SAE occurred and reported nausea and diarrhea were self-limiting [37]. More investigations and applications of this promising procedure are underway [38].

3.2 Gastric occupying devices

3.2.1 Transpyloric shuttle

The TransPyloric Shuttle (TPS) (BAROnova Goleta, CA, USA) is a gastric occupying device that is designed to delay gastric emptying and induce early and prolonged satiety [20]. The device consists of a spherical silicone orb that tapers into a tail tethered to a smaller cylindrical orb. After the device is delivered into the stomach through an overtube using a transluminal endoscopic procedure, the TPS moves freely in the stomach without the attachment to the tissue. Due to the physiological peristalsis, the small cylindrical orb will be pulled through the pylorus and reside in the duodenum. Because the base of the greater orb is compliant, it will self-position across the pylorus creating an intermittent seal intended to delay gastric emptying. Device removal is performed endoscopically, in which standard endoscopic graspers are used to unlock and retrieve the locking mechanism. Once unlocked, a standard endoscopic polypectomy snare can be used to retrieve the device.

3.2.1.1 Efficacy and safety profile

To date, only one feasibility study has investigated the safety and efficacy of the TPS [39]. Around 20 patients with a mean BMI of 36 kg/m^2 were randomized to TPS placement with treatment periods of either 3 or 6 months. Patients lost an average of 25.1 ± 14.0% of EWL in the 3-month group and those who had the device for 6 months lost an average of 41 ± 21.1%. Early device removal occurred in two patients because of acute onset of epigastric pain after 10.5 weeks and 5.5 months, respectively. After device removal, the complaints resolved immediately. No SAE were reported, and TPS insertion and removal procedures went without any problems. Gastric ulcer, localized in the antrum, occurred in 10 patients and was resolved by medication. The majority of adverse events reported were periprocedural and mild or moderate. However, the incidence of gastric ulcers prompted changes in the design of the TPS, with the new prototype now being studied in a multicenter randomized sham-controlled trial in the United States [40].

3.2.2 Full sense bariatric device

The Full Sense Bariatric Device (BKFW LLC, Grand rapids, MI, USA) is another gastric occupying device that comprises an esophageal stent connected to a gastric disk. It is hypothesized that it aids weight loss by placing direct and continuous pressure on the distal esophagus and cardia portion of the stomach, thereby inducing satiety. The pressure should provide continuous gastric nerve stimulation and hormonal feedback mechanisms that signals a feeling of fullness to the brain, even when there is no food present.

3.2.2.1 Efficacy and safety profile

In unpublished data with three human subjects, the device reportedly showed a 28% EWL after 46 days. During a 6-month trial in an unknown number of subjects, the device demonstrated a median EWL of 80%. However, no peer-reviewed data are currently available to determine its safety and efficacy [20].

4. Bariatric pacing and gastric electrical stimulation

4.1 Bariatric pacing

As early as 1980, the vagal system gained attention as a possible target in obesity treatment. Patients with peptic ulcer disease temporarily lost weight after truncal vagotomy [41, 42]. Only 10–20% of the vagal nerve fibers are composed of efferent fibers that control stomach activity, whereas the remaining 80–90% consist of afferent fibers that send signals regulating satiety and satiation [43]. With this in mind, application of electrical current to the stomach vagus nerve alters gastric myoelectrical activity. While the exact mechanism of action remains to be elucidated, bariatric pacing poses a new frontier in the treatment of severe obesity.

4.1.1 Maestro rechargeable system

Vagal blocking therapy (VBloc therapy) has been suggested as a new approach to tackle morbid obesity. Instead of performing a permanent truncal vagotomy, it blocks the vagal nerves in an intermittent manner using electrical pulses generated by the Maestro Rechargeable System (Enteromedics, St Paul, MN).

4.1.1.1 Technique

The maestro rechargeable system is an FDA approved implant device that is implanted with minimally invasive laparoscopic techniques. The system is provided with two leads which are placed around both the anterior and posterior vagal trunks at the level of the esophageal junction. Each lead delivers high-frequency, low energy, intermittent electrical pulses to its respective intra-abdominal vagal trunk for a predetermined period each day. This intermittent interruption of vagus nerve signaling leads to delayed gastric emptying which reduces feelings of hunger and promotes satiety [44]. A rechargeable neuroregulator is placed subcutaneously on the thoracic wall.

4.1.1.2 Efficacy and safety profile

Several feasibility studies have shown that VBloc therapy has a desirable safety profile and results in clinically important weight loss [45]. However, in the first randomized controlled trial comparing VBloc therapy with sham control, results were disappointing [46]. VBloc therapy was regarded safe, but weight loss was no greater in treated compared to control patients. Authors reported that the system electrical safety checks could have accounted for the weight loss in the control group. Another randomized controlled trial demonstrated 24.4% EWL in the VBloc group compared to 15.9% in the sham control group after a period of 12 months [47]. An open label follow-up study of the VBloc arm showed maintenance of weight loss in the majority of patients [48]. Adverse events were more frequently reported in the VBloc group and mostly involved heartburn or dyspepsia. Stronger evidence is needed to determine the place of VBloc therapy in the treatment of obesity.

4.2 Gastric electrical stimulation

Based on growing knowledge about gastrointestinal physiology, gastric electrical stimulation (GES) has been identified as a potential treatment modality for obesity [49, 50]. As early as 1995, the concept of GES was demonstrated in a series of animal experiments [51]. The exact mechanism of action of GES is still relatively unknown. However, it is thought that GES impairs gastric electrical activity, induces gastric distension, reduces gastric accommodation, and inhibits stomach peristalsis, thereby leading to delayed gastric emptying and increased satiety [52].

4.2.1 The transcend implantable gastric stimulator

A novel gastric electrical stimulator is the Transcend Implantable Gastric Stimulator (IGS, Transneuronix Inc., Mt Arlington, NJ, USA).

4.2.1.1 Technique

The device consists of one lead with two electrodes which is laparoscopically implanted on the lesser curvature near the pes anserinus and approximately 6 cm away from the pylorus. Proximally, the lead is fixed using an endostitch suture, and distally fixation is secured with the use of two clips. One electrode is positioned near the pes anserinus, while the other is placed near the esophagogastric junction. After adequate lead and electrode placement, the electrical pulse generator, which is connected to the lead, is implanted in a supra-fascial pocket and anchored with two sutures. Intraoperative gastroscopy is used to diagnose iatrogenic gastric perforation. After implantation, the device will be in off-mode for a period of 30 days, to allow the gastric tissue to heal before stimulation is initiated.

4.2.1.2 Efficacy and safety profile

A safety and feasibility study of the Transcend IGS implanted in 12 patients demonstrated a technically feasible and safe procedure [53]. In 25% of the patients, lead dislodgement occurred which required replacement. After 9 months, patients had lost a mean weight of 16 ± 12 kg. Another study conducted in 2002, in which 20 patients with a mean BMI of 40.9 kg/m^2 received the device, showed a % EWL of 10.6 ± 1.8 at 1 month, 1.5 ± 3.5 at 6 months, and 23.8 ± 5.0 at 10 months. Three intraoperative gastric penetrations were observed by gastroscopy. No further adverse events or complications were reported during the study period [54]. However, in a prospective double-blinded randomized sham-controlled trial, no difference was observed between the treatment and control group after a treatment period of 12 months [55]. Contributing to this was an investigator-initiated sub-study designed to assess whether IGS affects plasma levels of ghrelin and peptide YY which resulted in the conclusion that IGS does not prevent increase in fasting plasma levels of ghrelin that are associated with weight loss [56]. In conclusion, further studies are needed to determine whether changes in technology can provide meaningful weight loss and maintenance.

4.2.2 Tantalus gastric electrical stimulatory device

The Tantalus Electrical Stimulatory Device (Metacure, Israel) is a pulse generator accommodated with three bipolar leads. The device is designed to create an early activation of physiological satiety by enhancing physiological signals of gastric distensions and contractions. The system is capable of delivering gastric contractility modulation (GCM) signals triggered by food. The device senses spontaneous electrical activity of the smooth muscles and then delivers signals to enhance them. With the use of a specialized algorithm of electro-mechanical parameters in the gut, the system can detect the onset of a meal. It is hypothesized that enhancing of spontaneous gastric contractions in a very early stage of the meal, before reaching full gastric distension, induced early satiety by stimulation of stretch receptors. These elicit an increased input to the CNS, thereby promoting a feeling of fullness.

4.2.2.1 Technique

The system is implanted with the use of a laparoscope, whereby the three bipolar leads are placed in the sub-serosa of the gastric wall. One lead is placed in the fundus area to detect the intake of food, while the other two are positioned in the antrum for slow-wave detection and signal delivery. Nonabsorbable sutures and two clips are to ensure proper fixation at, respectively, the proximal and distal part of the lead. The procedure is carried out under both laparoscopic and gastroscopic visualization to prevent perforation of the gastric wall. After successful lead placement, the leads are connected to the implantable pulse generator which is placed in a subcutaneous pocket at the left side of the abdomen.

4.2.2.2 Efficacy and safety profile

In the first open-label single center trial, 12 patients with a mean BMI of 43.2 kg/m^2 underwent the implantation with the Tantalus system [57]. After 6 weeks of "off"-mode, the system got activated, which resulted in 17.6 ± 4.3% of EWL after a period of 20 weeks. Furthermore, a significant decrease in hunger, assessed with the three-factor eating questionnaire (TFEQ), was observed. Apart from two SAE including one case of rhabdomyolysis and one case of pulmonary embolism, the therapy was well tolerated. Both cases resolved completely without the need of surgical intervention, and patients were able to complete the study. In a study assessing the performance of the system, the algorithm was able to detect 73% of meals consumed with a false stimulation rate of 28% [58]. The majority of studies have also demonstrated a good improvement on glucose control in addition to weight loss [50, 59, 60].

5. Conclusion

New advancements in the field of bariatric endoscopy offer a promising entity to bridge the gap between lifestyle counseling, pharmaceutical treatment, and major surgical interventions in the treatment of obesity. Most of the procedures demonstrate the unique ability to be reversible or can be repeated throughout life for continued management of this disease. Besides, they have been proven to be not only effective in weight loss but also in the reduction of comorbidities associated with obesity. The results of these innovative techniques are very encouraging, and further clinical studies will likely occur in the near future. As we gain more evidence through well-designed conducted research, these treatment modalities can become an inherent part of everyday clinical practice.

Acknowledgements

We would like to thank Francisco Miguel Sánchez Margallo and his team for providing us with the opportunity to make a contribution to this chapter.

Conflict of interest

The author(s) declared no potential conflicts of interest with respect to the research, authorship, and/or publication of this chapter.

Author details

Suzanne Pruijssers*, Ernst van Heurn and Nicole Bouvy
Department of Surgery, Maastricht University Medical Center, Maastricht, The Netherlands

*Address all correspondence to: s.pruijssers@maastrichtuniversity.nl

References

[1] WHO. Obesity and Overweight Factsheet. 2018. Available from: http://www.who.int/news-room/fact-sheets/detail/obesity-and-overweight

[2] Ribaric G, Buchwald JN, McGlennon TW. Diabetes and weight in comparative studies of bariatric surgery vs conventional medical therapy: A systematic review and meta-analysis. Obesity Surgery. 2014;**24**(3):437-455

[3] Sjostrom L. Bariatric surgery and reduction in morbidity and mortality: Experiences from the SOS study. International Journal of Obesity. 2008;**32**(Suppl 7):S93-S97

[4] Ruban A, Ashrafian H, Teare JP. The EndoBarrier: Duodenal-jejunal bypass liner for diabetes and weight loss. Gastroenterology Research and Practice. 2018;**2018**:7823182

[5] Patel N, Mohanaruban A, Ashrafian H, Le Roux C, Byrne J, Mason J, et al. EndoBarrier(R): A safe and effective novel treatment for obesity and type 2 diabetes? Obesity Surgery. 2018;**28**(7):1980-1989

[6] Schouten R, Rijs CS, Bouvy ND, Hameeteman W, Koek GH, Janssen IM, et al. A multicenter, randomized efficacy study of the EndoBarrier Gastrointestinal Liner for presurgical weight loss prior to bariatric surgery. Annals of Surgery. 2010;**251**(2):236-243

[7] Koehestanie P, de Jonge C, Berends FJ, Janssen IM, Bouvy ND, Greve JW. The effect of the endoscopic duodenal-jejunal bypass liner on obesity and type 2 diabetes mellitus, a multicenter randomized controlled trial. Annals of Surgery. 2014;**260**(6):984-992

[8] Jirapinyo P, Haas AV, Thompson CC. Effect of the duodenal-jejunal bypass liner on glycemic control in patients with type 2 diabetes with obesity: A meta-analysis with secondary analysis on weight loss and hormonal changes. Diabetes Care. 2018;**41**(5):1106-1115

[9] Ryder REJ, Munro L, Mcmaster JJ, Bessell J, Bascomb JM, Collins JE, et al. First risk-benefit data from the worldwide endobarrier registry. Diabetes. 2018;**67**(Supplement 1)

[10] Forner PM, Ramacciotti T, Farey JE, Lord RV. Safety and effectiveness of an endoscopically placed duodenal-jejunal bypass device (EndoBarrier(R)): Outcomes in 114 patients. Obesity Surgery. 2017;**27**(12):3306-3313

[11] Quezada N, Munoz R, Morelli C, Turiel D, Hernandez J, Pimentel F, et al. Safety and efficacy of the endoscopic duodenal-jejunal bypass liner prototype in severe or morbidly obese subjects implanted for up to 3 years. Surgical Endoscopy. 2018;**32**(1):260-267

[12] Sandler BJ, Rumbaut R, Swain CP, Torres G, Morales L, Gonzales L, et al. Human experience with an endoluminal, endoscopic, gastrojejunal bypass sleeve. Surgical Endoscopy. 2011;**25**(9):3028-3033

[13] Sandler BJ, Rumbaut R, Swain CP, Torres G, Morales L, Gonzales L, et al. One-year human experience with a novel endoluminal, endoscopic gastric bypass sleeve for morbid obesity. Surgical Endoscopy. 2015;**29**(11):3298-3303

[14] Moreno C, Closset J, Dugardeyn S, Barea M, Mehdi A, Collignon L, et al. Transoral gastroplasty is safe, feasible, and induces significant weight loss in morbidly obese patients: Results of the second human pilot study. Endoscopy. 2008;**40**(5):406-413

[15] Deviere J, Ojeda Valdes G, Cuevas Herrera L, Closset J, Le Moine O, Eisendrath P, et al. Safety, feasibility and

weight loss after transoral gastroplasty: First human multicenter study. Surgical Endoscopy. 2008;**22**(3):589-598

[16] Familiari P, Costamagna G, Blero D, Le Moine O, Perri V, Boskoski I, et al. Transoral gastroplasty for morbid obesity: A multicenter trial with a 1-year outcome. Gastrointestinal Endoscopy. 2011;**74**(6):1248-1258

[17] Chiellini C, Iaconelli A, Familiari P, Riccioni ME, Castagneto M, Nanni G, et al. Study of the effects of transoral gastroplasty on insulin sensitivity and secretion in obese subjects. Nutrition, Metabolism, and Cardiovascular Diseases: NMCD. 2010;**20**(3):202-207

[18] Nanni G, Familiari P, Mor A, Iaconelli A, Perri V, Rubino F, et al. Effectiveness of the transoral endoscopic vertical gastroplasty (TOGa(R)): A good balance between weight loss and complications, if compared with gastric bypass and biliopancreatic diversion. Obesity Surgery. 2012;**22**(12):1897-1902

[19] Fayad L, Adam A, Dunlap M, Badurdeen DS, Hill C, Ajayi T, et al. Endoscopic sleeve gastroplasty versus laparoscopic sleeve gastrectomy: A case-matched study. Gastrointestinal Endoscopy. 2018

[20] Bazerbachi F, Vargas Valls EJ, Abu Dayyeh BK. Recent clinical results of endoscopic bariatric therapies as an obesity intervention. Clinical Endoscopy. 2017;**50**(1):42-50

[21] Jain D, Bhandari BS, Arora A, Singhal S. Endoscopic sleeve gastroplasty—A new tool to manage obesity. Clinical Endoscopy. 2017;**50**(6):552-561

[22] Graus Morales J, Crespo Perez L, Marques A, Marin Arribas B, Bravo Arribas R, Ramo E, et al. Modified endoscopic gastroplasty for the treatment of obesity. Surgical Endoscopy. 2018;**32**(9):3936-3942

[23] Lopez-Nava G, Sharaiha RZ, Vargas EJ, Bazerbachi F, Manoel GN, Bautista-Castano I, et al. Endoscopic sleeve gastroplasty for obesity: A multicenter study of 248 patients with 24 months follow-up. Obesity Surgery. 2017;**27**(10):2649-2655

[24] Sartoretto A, Sui Z, Hill C, Dunlap M, Rivera AR, Khashab MA, et al. Endoscopic sleeve gastroplasty (ESG) is a reproducible and effective endoscopic bariatric therapy suitable for widespread clinical adoption: A large, international multicenter study. Obesity Surgery. 2018;**28**(7):1812-1821

[25] Sharaiha RZ, Kumta NA, Saumoy M, Desai AP, Sarkisian AM, Benevenuto A, et al. Endoscopic sleeve gastroplasty significantly reduces body mass index and metabolic complications in obese patients. Clinical Gastroenterology and Hepatology. 2017;**15**(4):504-510

[26] Espinos JC, Turro R, Mata A, Cruz M, da Costa M, Villa V, et al. Early experience with the Incisionless Operating Platform (IOP) for the treatment of obesity: The Primary Obesity Surgery Endolumenal (POSE) procedure. Obesity Surgery. 2013;**23**(9):1375-1383

[27] Lopez-Nava G, Bautista-Castano I, Jimenez A, de Grado T, Fernandez-Corbelle JP. The Primary Obesity Surgery Endolumenal (POSE) procedure: One-year patient weight loss and safety outcomes. Surgery for Obesity and Related Diseases. 2015;**11**(4):861-865

[28] Miller K, Turro R, Greve JW, Bakker CM, Buchwald JN, Espinos JC. MILEPOST multicenter randomized controlled trial: 12-month weight loss and satiety outcomes after pose (SM) vs. medical therapy. Obesity Surgery. 2017;**27**(2):310-322

[29] Sullivan S, Swain JM, Woodman G, Antonetti M, De La Cruz-Munoz N, Jonnalagadda SS, et al. Randomized sham-controlled trial evaluating efficacy and safety of endoscopic gastric plication for primary obesity: The essential trial. Obesity. 2017;**25**(2):294-301

[30] DeAsis FJ, Denham W, Linn JG, Haggerty SP, Ujiki MB. Primary obesity surgery endoluminal. Surgical Endoscopy. 2017;**31**(2):951

[31] Espinos JC, Turro R, Moragas G, Bronstone A, Buchwald JN, Mearin F, et al. Gastrointestinal physiological changes and their relationship to weight loss following the POSE procedure. Obesity Surgery. 2016;**26**(5):1081-1089

[32] Huberty V, Ibrahim M, Hiernaux M, Chau A, Dugardeyn S, Deviere J. Safety and feasibility of an endoluminal-suturing device for endoscopic gastric reduction (with video). Gastrointestinal Endoscopy. 2017;**85**(4):833-837

[33] Huberty V, Machytka E, Boskoski I, Barea M, Costamagna G, Deviere J. Endoscopic gastric reduction with an endoluminal suturing device: A multicenter prospective trial with 1-year follow-up. Endoscopy. Dec 2018;**50**(12):1156-1162

[34] Verlaan T, Paulus GF, Mathus-Vliegen EMH, Veldhuyzen EAML, Conchillo JM, Bouvy ND, et al. Endoscopic gastric volume reduction with a novel articulating plication device is safe and effective in the treatment of obesity (with video). Gastrointestinal Endoscopy. 2015;**81**(2):312-320

[35] Machytka E, Buzga M, Ryou M, Lautz DB, Thompson CC. 1139 endoscopic dual-path enteral anastomosis using self-assembling magnets: First-in-human clinical feasibility. Gastroenterology. 2016;**150**(4):S232

[36] Machytka E, Buzga M, Lautz DB, Ryou M, Simonson D, Thompson CC. 103 A dual-path enteral bypass procedure created by a novel incisionless anastomosis system (IAS): 6-month clinical results. Gastroenterology. 2016;**150**(4):S26

[37] Machytka E, Buzga M, Zonca P, Lautz DB, Ryou M, Simonson DC, et al. Partial jejunal diversion using an incisionless magnetic anastomosis system: 1-year interim results in patients with obesity and diabetes. Gastrointestinal Endoscopy. 2017;**86**(5):904-912

[38] Vargas EJ, Rizk M, Bazerbachi F, Abu Dayyeh BK. Medical devices for obesity treatment: Endoscopic bariatric therapies. The Medical Clinics of North America. 2018;**102**(1):149-163

[39] Marinos G, Eliades C, Raman Muthusamy V, Greenway F. Weight loss and improved quality of life with a nonsurgical endoscopic treatment for obesity: Clinical results from a 3- and 6-month study. Surgery for Obesity and Related Diseases. 2014;**10**(5):929-934

[40] Sullivan S, Edmundowicz SA, Thompson CC. Endoscopic bariatric and metabolic therapies: New and emerging technologies. Gastroenterology. 2017;**152**(7):1791-1801

[41] Smith DK, Sarfeh J, Howard L. Truncal vagotomy in hypothalamic obesity. The Lancet. 1983;**1**(8337):1330-1331

[42] Kral JG. Vagotomy as a treatment for morbid obesity. The Surgical Clinics of North America. 1979;**59**(6):1131-1138

[43] Hwang SS, Takata MC, Fujioka K, Fuller W. Update on bariatric surgical procedures and an introduction to the implantable weight loss device: The maestro rechargeable system. Medical Devices. 2016;**9**:291-299

[44] Stimac D, Klobucar Majanovic S, Licina M. Recent trends in endoscopic

management of obesity. Surgical Innovation. 2016;**23**(5):525-537

[45] Camilleri M, Toouli J, Herrera MF, Kulseng B, Kow L, Pantoja JP, et al. Intra-abdominal vagal blocking (VBLOC therapy): Clinical results with a new implantable medical device. Surgery. 2008;**143**(6):723-731

[46] Sarr MG, Billington CJ, Brancatisano R, Brancatisano A, Toouli J, Kow L, et al. The EMPOWER study: Randomized, prospective, double-blind, multicenter trial of vagal blockade to induce weight loss in morbid obesity. Obesity Surgery. 2012;**22**(11):1771-1782

[47] Ikramuddin S, Blackstone RP, Brancatisano A, Toouli J, Shah SN, Wolfe BM, et al. Effect of reversible intermittent intra-abdominal vagal nerve blockade on morbid obesity: The ReCharge randomized clinical trial. Journal of the American Medical Association. 2014;**312**(9):915-922

[48] Apovian CM, Shah SN, Wolfe BM, Ikramuddin S, Miller CJ, Tweden KS, et al. Two-year outcomes of vagal nerve blocking (vBloc) for the treatment of obesity in the ReCharge trial. Obesity Surgery. 2017;**27**(1):169-176

[49] Greenway F, Zheng J. Electrical stimulation as treatment for obesity and diabetes. Journal of Diabetes Science and Technology. 2007;**1**(2):251-259

[50] Cha R, Marescaux J, Diana M. Updates on gastric electrical stimulation to treat obesity: Systematic review and future perspectives. World Journal of Gastrointestinal Endoscopy. 2014;**6**(9):419-431

[51] Cigaina VV, Pinato G, Rigo VV, Bevilacqua M, Ferraro F, Ischia S, et al. Gastric peristalsis control by mono situ electrical stimulation: A preliminary study. Obesity Surgery. 1996;**6**(3):247-249

[52] Chen J. Mechanisms of action of the implantable gastric stimulator for obesity. Obesity Surgery. 2004;**14** (Suppl 1):S28-S32

[53] D'Argent J. Gastric electrical stimulation as therapy of morbid obesity: Preliminary results from the French study. Obesity Surgery. 2002;**12**(Suppl 1):21s-25s

[54] Favretti F, De Luca M, Segato G, Busetto L, Ceoloni A, Magon A, et al. Treatment of morbid obesity with the transcend implantable gastric stimulator (IGS): A prospective survey. Obesity Surgery. 2004;**14**(5):666-670

[55] Shikora SA, Bergenstal R, Bessler M, Brody F, Foster G, Frank A, et al. Implantable gastric stimulation for the treatment of clinically severe obesity: Results of the SHAPE trial. Surgery for Obesity and Related Diseases. 2009;**5**(1):31-37

[56] Korner J, Nandi A, Wright SM, Waitman J, McMahon DJ, Bessler M, et al. Implantable gastric stimulator does not prevent the increase in plasma ghrelin levels that occurs with weight loss. Obesity. 2011;**19**(10):1935-1939

[57] Bohdjalian A, Prager G, Aviv R, Policker S, Schindler K, Kretschmer S, et al. One-year experience with Tantalus: A new surgical approach to treat morbid obesity. Obesity Surgery. 2006;**16**(5):627-634

[58] Policker S, Lu H, Haddad W, Aviv R, Kliger A, Glasberg O, et al. Electrical stimulation of the gut for the treatment of type 2 diabetes: The role of automatic eating detection. Journal of Diabetes Science and Technology. 2008;**2**(5):906-912

[59] Policker S, Haddad W, Yaniv I. Treatment of type 2 diabetes using meal-triggered gastric electrical stimulation. The Israel Medical Association Journal. 2009;**11**(4):206-208

[60] Sanmiguel CP, Conklin JL, Cunneen SA, Barnett P, Phillips EH, Kipnes M, et al. Gastric electrical stimulation with the TANTALUS system in obese type 2 diabetes patients: Effect on weight and glycemic control. Journal of Diabetes Science and Technology. 2009;**3**(4):964-970

Chapter 4

LaparoEndoscopic Single-Site Upper Gastrointestinal Surgery

Hytham K.S. Hamid and Sean M. Johnston

Abstract

The evolution of minimally invasive surgery has led to the development of laparoendoscopic single-site (LESS) surgery. The feasibility of almost all types of LESS upper (GI) procedures has been shown. During the learning phase, substantial experience in both laparoscopy and upper GI surgery and stringent patient selection criteria is essential for successful and safe application of the technique, especially in complex procedures. Comparative studies between LESS and conventional laparoscopy for various upper GI procedures suggest a non-inferiority of LESS over standard laparoscopy, although the only objective benefit remains an improved cosmetic outcome. Intracorporeal instrument collision, lack of triangulation, and in-line vision are among the main challenges of LESS surgery. The current review provides a comprehensive report of the specific applications of LESS in upper GI surgery, with a special reference to advances made to overcome the current technical difficulties and future perspectives.

Keywords: laparoendoscopic, laparoscopy, foregut, upper GI, cholecystectomy, ergonomics, single-port, single-incision

1. Introduction

Continued efforts to further reduce morbidity and improve the aesthetic outcomes of laparoscopic surgery while maintaining the same degree of safety and surgical efficiency have led to the evolution of single-port or single-incision laparoscopy. A surfeit of acronyms has been used to refer to these techniques until a consensus statement, following the first Laparoendoscopic Single-Site Surgery Consortium for Assessment and Research (LESSCAR), agreed to use the term "LESS" [1]. By reducing the number of transcutaneous points of access, the approach offers numerous advantages including but not limited to improving postoperative recovery time and pain, enhancing cosmesis, and minimizing port-related complications [2, 3].

2. Challenges, instrumentation, and techniques

Despite its early use in upper GI surgery, the LESS approach was slow to gain acceptance until recently, possibly due to technical difficulties, the need for specialized instruments, and the lack of clear benefits in comparison with conventional minimally invasive surgery. Close proximity of laparoscopic instruments and camera lens often results in intracorporeal instrument collision or "sword fighting", hindering the surgeon from operating dextrously within the operative field. Visibility of the operative field afforded by the camera assistant is also limited because of the restriction in freedom to manoeuvre the camera lens to minimize instrument clashing. Moreover, intracorporeal dissection and suturing are challenging because of the limited range of movement of the laparoscopic instruments working along the same axis with lack of triangulation [3, 4].

Several techniques and advancements have been introduced to overcome constraints associated with LESS approach. New access devices have been designed and commercialized and are chosen according to the discretion of the surgeons in each institute. The most commonly used are multichannel single-port devices (e.g. Quad Port®, Tri Port®, SILS Port®) or single-channel devices in which multiple trocars can be placed (e.g. GelPOINT® and SSL port®) [5]. There are also devices of art which allow the use of items in the operating room, such as surgical glove with adaptation of trocars in each finger [6].

Another important advance in the development of LESS surgery was the appearance of modified curved instruments, articulated and reusable pre-bent, which provide better force application at instrument tip during dissection and improved intraoperative ergonomics [7]. Needlescopic instruments have been rediscovered, as they can be introduced through a small puncture that requires no formal closure [8, 9]. Low-profile camera systems and laparoscopes with high definition and flexible tip options (e.g. ENDOEYE® and Ideal Eyes®) have also been developed to reduce crowding with other instruments and improve visualization [5]. Additionally, instruments clashing can further be ameliorated by the cross-hand technique, which allows surgeons to manipulate instruments in a more intuitive way [10].

Finally, the need for a retraction mechanism that does not require an additional port led to the development of several techniques and manoeuvres such as patient repositioning and utilization of gravity and insertion of gauze between surgical planes [11, 12]. Other procedure-specific manoeuvres for internal retraction are discussed in the relevant sections.

3. Specific LESS applications in upper GI surgery

The application of LESS approach in upper GI surgery was first described in 1997 by Navarra et al. who reported a series of 30 cases of LESS cholecystectomy performed via a single umbilical incision [13]. Subsequently, many clinical series and randomized controlled trials (RCTs) have been reported, and almost the entire spectrum of surgical procedures for upper GI tract diseases has been described and shown to be feasible.

3.1 LESS gastric surgery

3.1.1 LESS gastrectomy

Since the first description by Omori et al. in 2011 [14], only few case series have been published on LESS gastrectomy for gastric tumours, mostly from Korea and Japan [11]. *All these series* have reported techniques and outcomes of LESS distal gastrectomy, while LESS total and proximal gastrectomy and LESS wedge resection have only been reported as individual cases [15–18]. This is because the procedure is complex and technically difficult to perform, and there are concerns regarding oncologic safety. Favourable factors for performing LESS distal gastrectomy include previous experience with conventional multiport laparoscopic gastrectomy and low patient BMI [19].

3.1.1.1 Technical considerations

In early experiences with the technique, additional needlescopic instruments were required outside of the single incision [14, 20]. For pure LESS distal gastrectomy, the access is transumbilical, and a percutaneous suture is often used for liver retraction. Gastric mobilization, lymph node dissection, and reconstruction are generally performed in the same manner as in conventional laparoscopic distal gastrectomy with few modifications. In performing LESS D2 gastrectomy, the suprapancreatic lymph node dissection, especially station 11p, can be technically challenging because it lies behind the pancreas and is vertical to the direction of instruments, and some authors recommend incomplete safe exploration [21]. Alternatively, mid-pancreas mobilization and traction have been described to achieve complete dissection of station 11p lymph nodes without assistance [22]. Billroth II and extracorporeal or intracorporeal uncut Roux-en Y gastrojejunostomy remain the most commonly used methods for reconstruction in pure LESS distal gastrectomy [21, 23]. Recently, unaided delta-shaped (uDelta) gastroduodenostomy has been introduced as a modification of the original advanced assistance-dependent delta-shaped anastomosis, which is considered a safe and more reproducible reconstruction option, with similar anatomical results [24].

3.1.1.2 Outcomes

Comparative series between conventional multiport laparoscopy and LESS approach for distal gastrectomy have recently been reported. These studies demonstrated comparable outcomes in terms of operative time, conversion, postoperative mortality, lymph node harvest, R0 resection, and 5-year overall and disease-free survival between the two groups, illustrating the safety and feasibility of LESS distal gastrectomy for both early and advanced gastric cancer [25–28]. Conversely, while no significant differences in the postoperative complications were noted between the two approaches in patients with early gastric cancer [25, 26], the overall complication rate was significantly lower after LESS distal gastrectomy for advanced gastric cancer [28]. Pointing to faster recovery, studies evidenced earlier initiation of oral intake, lower pain scores on postoperative day 0 and 1, less analgesics requirements, and shorter hospital stay for the LESS approach than the conventional laparoscopic counterpart [26–28]. Only one study evaluated the cosmetic outcomes using the numerical rating scale assessment of the scar and reported more satisfaction in the LESS group [26].

In a separate analysis, when reduced-port laparoscopic and LESS distal gastrectomy for early gastric cancer were compared, no significant differences were observed in the perioperative and oncologic outcomes. However, there were more females and nonobese patients in the LESS group [29]. Recently, Suh et al. reported the results of 16 patients who underwent LESS distal gastrectomy with uDelta gastroduodenostomy or uncut Roux-en Y gastrojejunostomy. There were no significant differences in mean operative time, transfusion rates, hospitalization, anastomosis-related complications, and 30-day mortality. Interestingly, the reconstruction time for uDelta was shorter than that for Roux-en Y anastomosis [24].

3.1.2 LESS intragastric surgery

LESS intragastric resection is a novel approach that has mainly been employed in the management of gastric stromal tumours, although its use for gastric bezoar removal has been described [30]. The procedure is particularly useful in cases of endophytic tumours <5 cm, with unfavourable locations, such as the fundus, high lying in the posterior wall of the stomach, or close to the gastroesophageal junction or the pyloric ring [31–33]. Several advantages are offered by the LESS intragastric approach including direct visualization of tumours during resection, minimal dissemination of the tumour into the peritoneal cavity, easy delivery of the specimen through the single-site incision, and extracorporeal repair of the gastrotomy site [31]. In addition, it obviates the need for multiple incisions, thus resulting in better cosmesis, and reduces the possibility of deformity by significantly preserving the normal gastric tissue with more precise resection compared with conventional laparoscopic wedge resection [33].

3.1.2.1 Technical considerations

LESS intragastric resection may be performed either as a "pure" LESS procedure or less commonly as a "hybrid" procedure with intraoperative gastroscopy [33, 34]. Both umbilical and left upper quadrant incision can be used to obtain access to the peritoneal cavity. A 2–3 cm incision is performed on the anterior wall or the lower body greater curvature of the stomach, and a single multichannel port or three standard ports are inserted through the abdominal incision and gastrotomy site [32, 33]. After creating a pneumostomach, the tumour is located, excised, and retrieved through the single-site incision.

3.1.2.2 Outcomes

Despite the small number of cases reported in the literature, the procedure appears to be safe and effective, with favourable outcomes. In previous series, no conversion to conventional laparoscopy or open surgery was necessary nor were additional trocars. Postoperative complications occurred in 0–25% and were mostly intragastric and surgical site bleeding [31, 32, 35, 36]. The operative time, number of used staplers, time to first oral intake, hospital stay, and complications were not significantly different from conventional laparoscopic wedge resection [33]. No local recurrence or distant metastasis was detected during a follow-up period of 8–19 months [31–33].

3.2 LESS hepatobiliary surgery

3.2.1 LESS hepatic surgery

The first report of LESS hepatectomy was published by Aldrighetti et al. in 2010. The authors performed a left lateral sectionectomy via a supraumbilical incision for a solitary colorectal metastasis [37]. Nonetheless, because LESS liver resection requires advanced surgical skills and has a significant learning curve, only a limited number of reports are currently available in the literature. The procedure has been used for wide range of conditions: liver adenoma, focal nodular hyperplasia, haemangioma, hydatid and simple cyst, intrahepatic biliary stones, metastatic liver lesions, and hepatocellular carcinoma [38].

Patients should be cautiously selected for LESS liver resection. Superficial hepatic lesions limited to the left lateral section are preferable, even though bigger or more technically challenging resections for less favourably located tumours have been described with increased experience in the technique [39]. Lesions less than 5 and 10 cm are the recommended cut-off points for malignant and benign tumours, respectively [39]. Other contraindications include vascular or extrahepatic involvement and morbid obesity [40–42].

3.2.1.1 Technical considerations

Transumbilical incision with a 3-trocar technique has been the preferred approach; right upper quadrant or supraumbilical incisions can be useful in the setting of portal hypertension with umbilical varices or lesions in distant segments [43, 44]. Several methods were adopted to avoid instrument collision including the use of single ports with a large outer cap or self-retaining sleeves [38]. During parenchymal dissection, simultaneous in-line radiofrequency precoagulation can be used to reduce the risk of bleeding [45]. Similar to other foregut procedure, the resection specimen is placed into a retrieval bag prior to removal through the port site.

3.2.1.2 Outcomes

Benzing et al. recently performed a comprehensive systematic review on LESS hepatectomy pooling the available data of 124 minor and 7 major resections of 133 patients from 15 studies [46]. The majority of minor resections were left lateral sectionectomies and wedge resections for both benign and malignant diseases; 6 of the 7 major resections were performed due to malignancy, including 4 for colorectal metastasis. Overall, the conversion to multiport laparoscopic/open rate ranged between 0 and 25% which, for the most part, was due to technical difficulties, intraoperative bleeding, and uncertainty of the oncologic margin of the resection. Free resection margins could be achieved in all but one patient with malignancy, demonstrating the efficacy of the technique. The median length of hospital stay was reported between 1 and 21 days, and the overall morbidity and mortality rates were 6.8% (0–33%) and 0.8%, respectively [46].

Few studies have compared the outcomes of LESS and conventional laparoscopic left lateral liver sectionectomy, and the results were inconclusive or conflicting. Including only patients with benign liver diseases, an RCT demonstrated a significantly shorter length of hospital stay in the LESS group [47]. This difference, however, disappeared in the other two non-randomized matched and unmatched comparisons, when patients with malignant tumours were also included [48, 49]. A further advantage observed only by Struecker et al. for the LESS technique was shorter operative time, which was attributed to the easy retrieval of the specimen through the umbilical incision [49]. The intraoperative blood loss, conversion, and postoperative morbidity and analgesics requirements were similar between the two groups in all studies. It was indicated that in well-selected patients with either benign or malignant hepatic lesions, LESS left lateral sectionectomy can provide a safe and effective alternative to multiport laparoscopic surgery [47–49].

Choi et al. described the surgical outcomes of LESS- and standard laparoscopy-assisted donor right hepatectomy. The LESS group had significantly shorter operative time, less blood loss, earlier resumption of enteral feeding, and lower pain scores. There were no significant differences between the groups with respect to length of hospital stay, R0 resection, and postoperative morbidity and mortality [50]. These results were replicated by Han et al. who described the surgical outcomes of LESS and conventional laparoscopic method for major and minor hepatectomies. Nevertheless, in this retrospective study, patient background and the type of procedures differed between the two groups, meaning the analysis was constrained by selection bias [51].

3.2.2 LESS cholecystectomy

The LESS approach has been increasingly used in gallbladder surgery, and its indications are expanding by virtue of the advances in instrumentation and surgical experience. Over the last two decades, hundreds of studies have been published reporting outcomes of LESS cholecystectomy and describing different operative techniques for the procedure with variable success rates [52].

3.2.2.1 Technical considerations

The access to the peritoneal cavity in LESS cholecystectomy is obtained through paraumbilical or more commonly intraumbilical incision, which, although provides the best cosmetic outcome, is associated with higher rates of wound complications and incisional hernia [52]. A single 20–30 mm fasciotomy incision with a reusable or disposable single-access device can be used. "Swiss cheese" technique, a multiple facia puncture technique using multiple low-profile ports, is an acceptable alternative though carries risk of air leak and facial weakness [52, 53]. Various types of instruments have been used in LESS cholecystectomy including standard straight and curved instruments, with the latter offers the advantage of triangulation within the operative field [53]. During dissection, several technical variations are adopted to achieve adequate gallbladder anchorage and a clear critical view of safety while obviating the necessity of an extra port: suture suspension ("puppet technique"), internal retraction, transabdominal endoloop, and magnet grasper [54]. Gallbladder is thereafter delivered through a single-access device or connected facial openings with or without the use of a retrieval bag.

3.2.2.2 Outcomes

Several meta-analyses have compared the outcomes of LESS cholecystectomy with traditional multiport (three or four ports) laparoscopic cholecystectomy [55–66]. Although early reports showed no significant differences in terms of reported pain and quantity of on-demand analgesics delivered, the three most recent meta-analyses included more RCTs with different inclusion criteria and showed less postoperative pain following LESS cholecystectomy particularly in the first 24 h [64–66]. This discrepancy in results is possibly ascribable to the less tissue trauma in LESS cholecystectomy as surgeons progress along the learning curve and gain experience with the technique. The operative time was significantly longer in the LESS group in all meta-analyses, whereas open conversion rate and length of hospital stay were nearly identical between the two groups. Conversion to multiport and/or open cholecystectomy in the LESS group was mainly due to omental adhesions, obesity, Mirizzi syndrome, and obscure anatomy of Calot's triangle [59, 62]. Of note, the overall short-term postoperative morbidity rate, surgical site infection, and port-site hernia were consistently higher, though not statistically significant, in the LESS group than the conventional group [55–65]. This was further bolstered by a recent large pooled analysis indicating that mild and severe adverse events were significantly higher in LESS cholecystectomy than in conventional laparoscopic cholecystectomy. When the results were adjusted to the type of technique used (4-port or 3-port), statistically significant differences were still noted [66]. Possible explanation of this raised risk of complications is the impaired exposure of the operative field in LESS cholecystectomy and the technical difficulty encountered by surgeons early during their learning phase. Moreover, the natural progression of this new technique to broader indications such as acute cholecystitis entails higher rates of adverse events.

Compared to conventional cholecystectomy, the inherent benefits of the LESS technique, specifically postoperative satisfaction and cosmetic outcomes, were significantly in favour of LESS cholecystectomy at different time points during the first postoperative year, which was at the expense of higher surgery costs. These results were replicated in most RCTs and all pooled analyses regardless of the scoring system employed: visual analogue scale (VAS), body image and cosmesis (BIQ), cosmesis, and wound satisfaction scores [56–66]. Meanwhile, apart from marginal advantage of LESS cholecystectomy early in the postoperative course, studies could not demonstrate any significant differences in the quality of life between LESS and conventional laparoscopic cholecystectomy in the first 12 months postoperatively [58, 63–66]. It is noteworthy to mention that despite the evidence for better patients' satisfaction and cosmetic results in LESS cholecystectomy, cosmetic outcome is not the main factor that drives patient preference. Rather the risk of complications seems to exercise a higher influence on patients in determining the choice of procedure [67]. This indicates that an improved postoperative morbidity rate is a prerequisite for LESS cholecystectomy to become widely accepted.

3.2.3 LESS common bile duct exploration

While the past decade has seen a dramatic increase in the adoption of LESS technique in gallbladder surgery, technical limitations have restricted its use in bile duct surgery to only highly selected cases. LESS exploration of the common bile duct (CBD) allows for combined treatment of cholelithiasis and choledocholithiasis using cholecystectomy and CBD drainage, a one-stage minimally invasive procedure with cosmetic advantage. At present, only a few case series of LESS CBD exploration have been reported in the literature, using either a single multichannel port or multiple trocars through a single intraumbilical or paraumbilical incision. Both transcystic and choledochotomy approaches with or without the assistance of a needlescopic grasper have been employed in LESS CBD exploration with successful ductal clearance rates ranging between 75 and 100%; conversion to open and conventional laparoscopic surgery was reported in 0–7.7% and 0–8.3%, respectively, and postoperative complications occurred in 0–25% [68–72]. Furthermore, Chuang et al. described a novel LESS transfistulous bile duct exploration and stone removal without drainage for Mirizzi syndrome type II with 80% success rate [73]. Supporting previous results and adding more evidence to the safety of the technique, the same authors reported 101 consecutive cases of successful LESS CBD exploration and concluded that in experienced hands, the procedure is feasible and a safe option for treatment of complicated and noncomplicated choledocholithiasis under low threshold for conversion [74].

In a series comparing 17 LESS and 17 conventional laparoscopic cholecystectomy and CBD exploration, Kim and colleagues reported (the study evidenced) a longer operating time in the LESS cohort but with less analgesics requirement and a shorter hospital stay. The stone clearance rate (100%) and incidence of complications were similar between the two groups [71]. A subsequent similar analysis by Chuang et al. did not show any significant difference in the operative outcomes between LESS and conventional laparoscopic CBD exploration. The former group however had a significantly higher rate of acute cholecystitis than the latter group, and this may have influenced the results [72].

3.3 LESS pancreatic surgery

The application of LESS approach to pancreatic surgery still remains an open debate. This procedure is generally considered as technically demanding due to its complexity and the need to perform fine dissections in a narrow surgical space. Indications for LESS pancreatic surgery include splenic artery aneurysm, pancreatic fibrosis, cysts, and benign and malignant neoplasms [12, 75]. The most commonly performed procedure is LESS distal pancreatectomy with or without spleen preservation for localized lesions; others include pancreatic necrosectomy and staging laparoscopy for advanced pancreatic cancer [76, 77].

3.3.1 Technical considerations

The approach in LESS distal pancreatectomy is mostly transumbilical. Occasionally, an additional 5 mm trocar is inserted in the left upper quadrant to be used by the surgeon's right hand and subsequently for drainage [78]. Various modifications of gastric suspension technique have been developed to facilitate better exposure of the pancreas [79–81]. The Lasso technique, in which a ribbon tape is looped around the pancreas body or tail, can be used to provide additional traction, particularly in cases of LESS distal pancreatectomy without splenic preservation [81, 82]. The pancreatic mobilization and dissection follow the principles of standard laparoscopic pancreatic resection, and the resected specimen is extracted through the umbilical site.

3.3.2 Outcomes

In a recent review, Chatzizacharias et al. analysed the data on LESS distal pancreatectomy from eight case studies. Conversion to open rate was 0–19%, and postoperative complications, mainly pancreatic fistula, were reported in 22% (0–50%) of patients. The length of hospital stay ranged between 1 and 15 days [39].

More importantly, Han et al. compared the outcomes between patients undergoing LESS and conventional laparoscopic distal pancreatectomy. With the exception of significantly longer operative time and duration of hospital stay reported with the LESS approach, perioperative outcomes did not differ between the two groups [83]. Likewise, two comparative analyses, including a case-control study, yielded no significant differences between conventional laparoscopic and LESS distal pancreatectomy in the operative time, intraoperative bleeding, conversion rate, resection status, hospital stay, and complications [75, 84]. The spleen was preserved more in the conventional group than in the LESS group, but this difference was not significant [83, 84]. A recent comparison between LESS and the more widely accepted robotic distal pancreatectomy has evidenced a significantly longer operative time and hospital stay, larger intraoperative blood loss, less spleen preservation, and higher grade II/IIIa postoperative complications in the LESS group. There were no significant differences in pain scores, tumour size, conversion rate, and overall complications between the two groups [85]. Overall, although it has been shown to be safe and feasible, these findings highlight the question of any real value of LESS approach in the context of pancreatic surgery.

3.4 LESS splenic surgery

Despite the scarcity of high-level evidence, there has been a dramatic increase in the number of laparoscopic splenectomies performed over the last 2 decades. The procedure is currently considered the gold standard for management of surgical diseases in normal or slightly enlarged spleens [86]. More recently, and as a bridging procedure towards pure natural orifice transluminal endoscopic surgery, Barbaros and Dinççağ were the first to describe LESS splenectomy in two female patients with idiopathic thrombocytopenic purpura [87]. Other common indications for this approach are splenic cystic disease, hereditary spherocytosis, myeloproliferative disorder, and splenic aneurysms and neoplasms [88].

3.4.1 Technical considerations

For LESS splenectomy, either a transumbilical or a lateral rectus incision can be utilized depending on the size of spleen. The technique used for splenic dissection is similar to multiport laparoscopic splenectomy. Not uncommonly, a 3 mm instrument is inserted through the left flank to facilitate spleen retraction and dissection of retroperitoneal adhesions [89]. Others used a cloth tape to encircle and tug the splenic hilum, therefore providing better exposure and easy introduction of the stapler into the splenic hilum [90]. Once the spleen is completely free, an endobag is deployed, and the spleen is retrieved intact or morcellated.

3.4.2 Outcomes

A systematic review published by Fan et al. summarized the evidence on LESS splenectomy from 29 articles, with a total of 105 patients. The median length of hospital stay varied from 1 to 11 days. The postoperative complication rate was 0–33.3%, and the rates of conversion to open and multiport laparoscopic surgery were 1.9 and 2.9%, respectively. Bleeding from the splenic or short gastric vessels were the main reasons for conversion. No perioperative death was observed [88]. In a comparison between reduced-port, multiport, and LESS splenectomy, Monclova et al. reported significantly longer operative time in the LESS group, and this was partly related to the higher spleen weight. Importantly, there was a significant advantage in the LESS and reduced-port groups in the body image index with respect to the multiport group, pointing to better cosmetic outcome. Other perioperative outcomes were comparable among the two groups [91]. Wu et al. conducted a comprehensive meta-analysis comparing the outcomes of LESS and conventional laparoscopic splenectomies. They pooled and meta-analysed the data of 332 patients from nine comparative and one prospective case-control study. While postoperative pain scores favoured the LESS approach, the conversion rate and operative time slightly favoured conventional laparoscopic surgery, though without statistical significance. Ultimately, no differences were observed with regard to morbidity, mortality, analgesics requirements, and postoperative hospitalization. The authors pointed out that LESS splenectomy is safe and feasible with no obvious advantages over multiport laparoscopic splenectomy [92].

4. Conclusions

The current evidence shows that LESS upper GI surgery is feasible, and its adoption is expanding worldwide. A successful LESS procedure requires proper instrumentation, adequate laparoscopic experience, and careful patient selection. The demonstration of a significant and consistent increase in the adverse events associated with certain LESS applications in upper GI surgery should represent a word of caution in performing these procedures. While cosmetic improvement is a natural corollary to LESS, real advantages of the approach in upper GI surgery are still controversial. Prospective randomized studies are largely awaited to further explore the benefits of this technique for patients as well as to elucidate the cost-effectiveness of the approach. The advent of new instruments and platforms may significantly counteract technical issues associated with LESS surgery and facilitates the current steep learning curve.

Conflict of interest

The authors declare no conflict of interest.

Author details

Hytham K.S. Hamid[1*] and Sean M. Johnston[2]

1 Soba University Hospital, Khartoum, Sudan

2 Tullamore Regional Hospital, Tullamore, Ireland

*Address all correspondence to: kujali2@gmail.com

References

[1] Gill IS, Advincula AP, Aron M, et al. Consensus statement of the consortium for laparoendoscopic single-site surgery. Surgical Endoscopy. 2010;**24**:762-768. DOI: 10.1007/s00464-009-0688-8

[2] Evans L, Manley K. Is there a cosmetic advantage to single-incision laparoscopic surgical techniques over standard laparoscopic surgery? A systematic review and meta-analysis. Surgical Laparoscopy, Endoscopy & Percutaneous Techniques. 2016;**26**(3):177-182. DOI: 10.1097/SLE.0000000000000261

[3] Ahmed I, Paraskeva P. A clinical review of single-incision laparoscopic surgery. The Surgeon. 2011;**9**(6):341-351. DOI: 10.1016/j.surge.2011.06.003

[4] Goel R, Lomanto D. Controversies in single-port laparoscopic surgery. Surgical Laparoscopy, Endoscopy & Percutaneous Techniques. 2012;**22**(5):380-382. DOI: 10.1097/SLE.0b013e3182615776

[5] Tsai AY, Selzer DJ. Single-port laparoscopic surgery. Advances in Surgery. 2010;**44**:1-27

[6] Livraghi L, Berselli M, Bianchi V, Latham L, Farassino L, Cocozza E. Glove technique in single-port access laparoscopic surgery: Results of an initial experience. Minimally Invasive Surgery. 2012;**2012**:415430. DOI: 10.1155/2012/415430

[7] Rao PP, Rao PP, Bhagwat S. Single-incision laparoscopic surgery—Current status and controversies. Journal of Minimal Access Surgery. 2011;7(1):6-16. DOI: 10.4103/0972-9941.72360

[8] Kim TS, Kim KH, An CH, Kim JS. Single center experiences of needle-scopic grasper assisted single incision laparoscopic cholecystectomy for gallbladder benign disease: Comparison with conventional 3-port laparoscopic cholecystectomy. Annals of Surgical Treatment and Research. 2016;**91**(5):233-238. DOI: 10.4174/astr.2016.91.5.233

[9] Palanivelu P, Patil KP, Parthasarathi R, Viswambharan JK, Senthilnathan P, Palanivelu C. Review of various liver retraction techniques in single incision laparoscopic surgery for the exposure of hiatus. Journal of Minimal Access Surgery. 2015;**11**(3):198-202. DOI: 10.4103/0972-9941.140202

[10] Ishikawa N, Arano Y, Shimizu S, Morishita M, Kawaguchi M, Matsunoki A, et al. Single incision laparoscopic surgery (SILS) using cross hand technique. Minimally Invasive Therapy & Allied Technologies. 2009;**18**(6):322-324. DOI: 10.3109/13645700903384492

[11] Lee Y, Kim HH. Single-incision laparoscopic gastrectomy for gastric cancer. Journal of Gastric Cancer. 2017;**17**(3):193-203. DOI: 10.5230/jgc.2017.17.e29

[12] Wang K, Fan Y. Minimally invasive distal pancreatectomy: Review of the English literature. Journal of Laparoendoscopic & Advanced Surgical Techniques. Part A. 2017;**27**(2):134-140. DOI: 10.1089/lap.2016.0132

[13] Navarra G, Pozza E, Occhionorelli S, Carcoforo P, Donini I. One wound laparoscopic cholecystectomy. The British Journal of Surgery. 1997;**84**:695

[14] Omori T, Oyama T, Akamatsu H, Tori M, Ueshima S, Nishida T. Transumbilical single-incision laparoscopic distal gastrectomy for early gastric cancer. Surgical Endoscopy. 2011;**25**:2400-2404. DOI: 10.1007/s00464-010-1563-3

[15] Lee CM, Park DW, Jung DH, Jang YJ, Kim JH, Park S, et al. Single-port

laparoscopic proximal gastrectomy with double tract reconstruction for early gastric cancer: Report of a case. Journal of Gastric Cancer. 2016;**16**:200-206. DOI: 10.5230/jgc.2016.16.3.200

[16] Ahn SH, Son SY, Jung DH, Park YS, Shin DJ, Park DJ, et al. Solo intracorporeal esophagojejunostomy reconstruction using a laparoscopic scope holder in single-port laparoscopic total gastrectomy for early gastric cancer. Journal of Gastric Cancer. 2015;**15**:132-138. DOI: 10.5230/jgc.2015.15.2.132

[17] Ertem M, Ozveri E, Gok H, Ozben V. Single incision laparoscopic total gastrectomy and d2 lymph node dissection for gastric cancer using a four-access single port: The first experience. Case Reports in Surgery. 2013;**2013**:504549. DOI: 10.1155/2013/504549

[18] Sasaki A, Koeda K, Obuchi T, Nakajima J, Nishizuka S, Terashima M, et al. Tailored laparoscopic resection for suspected gastric gastrointestinal stromal tumors. Surgery. 2010;**147**(4):516-520. DOI: 10.1016/j.surg.2009.10.035

[19] Lee B, Lee YT, Park YS, Ahn SH, Park DJ, Kim HH. Learning curve of pure single-port laparoscopic distal gastrectomy for gastric cancer. Journal of Gastric Cancer. 2018;**18**(2):182-188. DOI: 10.5230/jgc.2018.18.e20

[20] Park DJ, Lee JH, Ahn SH, Eng AK, Kim HH. Single-port laparoscopic distal gastrectomy with D1+β lymph node dissection for gastric cancers: Report of 2 cases. Surgical Laparoscopy, Endoscopy & Percutaneous Techniques. 2012;**22**:e214-e216. DOI: 10.1097/SLE.0b013e318253df9b

[21] Suh YS, Lee HJ, Yang HK. Single incision gastrectomy for gastric cancer. Translational Gastroenterology and Hepatology. 2016;**1**:41. DOI: 10.21037/tgh.2016.05.05

[22] Ahn SH, Jung Do H, Son SY, Park Do J, Kim HH. Pure single-incision laparoscopic D2 lymphadenectomy for gastric cancer: A novel approach to 11p lymph node dissection (midpancreas mobilization). Annals of Surgical Treatment and Research. 2014;**87**:279-283. DOI: 10.4174/astr.2014.87.5.279

[23] Inaki N. Reduced port laparoscopic gastrectomy: A review, techniques, and perspective. Asian Journal of Endoscopic Surgery. 2015;**8**(1):1-10. DOI: 10.1111/ases.12163

[24] Suh YS, Park JH, Kim TH, Huh YJ, Son YG, Yang JY, et al. Unaided stapling technique for pure single-incision distal gastrectomy in early gastric cancer: Unaided delta-shaped anastomosis and uncut Roux-en-Y anastomosis. Journal of Gastric Cancer. 2015;**15**:105-112. DOI: 10.5230/jgc.2015.15.2

[25] Zhou J, He Q, Wang J, Liu Q, Wang M. Application of enhanced recovery after surgery in single-incision laparoscopic distal gastrectomy. Surgical Laparoscopy, Endoscopy & Percutaneous Techniques. 2017;**27**(6):449-455. DOI: 10.1097/SLE.0000000000000474

[26] Ahn SH, Son SY, Jung DH, Park DJ, Kim HH. Pure single-port laparoscopic distal gastrectomy for early gastric cancer: Comparative study with multi-port laparoscopic distal gastrectomy. Journal of the American College of Surgeons. 2014;**219**:933-943. DOI: 10.1016/j.jamcollsurg.2014.07.009

[27] Omori T, Fujiwara Y, Moon J, Sugimura K, Miyata H, Masuzawa T, et al. Comparison of single-incision and conventional multi-port laparoscopic distal gastrectomy with D2 lymph node dissection for gastric cancer: A propensity score-matched analysis. Annals of Surgical Oncology.

2016;**23**:817-824. DOI: 10.1245/s10434-016-5485-8

[28] Omori T, Fujiwara Y, Yamamoto K, Yanagimoto Y, Sugimura K, Masuzawa T, et al. The safety and feasibility of single-port laparoscopic gastrectomy for advanced gastric cancer. Journal of Gastrointestinal Surgery. 5 Sept 2018. DOI: 10.1007/s11605-018-3937-0

[29] Kim SM, Ha MH, Seo JE, Kim JE, Choi MG, Sohn TS, et al. Comparison of single-port and reduced-port totally laparoscopic distal gastrectomy for patients with early gastric cancer. Surgical Endoscopy. 2016;**30**:3950-3957. DOI: 10.1007/s00464-015-4706-8

[30] Son T, Inaba K, Woo Y, Pak KH, Hyung WJ, Noh SH. New surgical approach for gastric bezoar: "Hybrid access surgery" combined intragastric and single port surgery. Journal of Gastric Cancer. 2011;**11**(4):230-233. DOI: 10.5230/jgc.2011.11.4.230

[31] Na J-U, Lee S-I, Noh S-M. The single incision laparoscopic intragastric wedge resection of gastric submucosal tumor. Journal of Gastric Cancer. 2011;**11**(4):225-229. DOI: 10.5230/jgc.2011.11.4.225

[32] DE Vogelaere K, VAN DE Winkel N, Simoens C, Delvaux G. Intragastric SILS for GIST, a new challenge in oncologic surgery: First experiences. Anticancer Research. 2013;**33**(8):3359-3363

[33] Choi CI, Lee SH, Hwang SH, Kim DH, Jeon TY, Kim DH, et al. Various features of laparoscopic tailored resection for gastric submucosal tumours: A single institution's results for 168 patients. Surgical Endoscopy. 2016;**30**(4):1450-1458. DOI: 10.1007/s00464-015-4350-3

[34] Cazauran JB, Mercier F, Pasquer A, Dominici P, Cotte E, Vaudoyer D, et al. Intragastric single-incision laparoscopic surgery for gastric leiomyoma: A stepwise approach. Annals of Surgical Oncology. 2017;**24**(8):2281. DOI: 10.1245/s10434-017-5868-5

[35] Choi CI, Lee SH, Hwang SH, Kim DH, Jeon TY, Kim DH, et al. Single-incision intragastric resection for upper and mid gastric submucosal tumours: A case-series study. Annals of Surgical Treatment and Research. 2014;**87**(6):304-310. DOI: 10.4174/astr.2014.87.6.304

[36] Katsuyama S, Nakajima K, Kurokawa Y, Takahashi T, Miyazaki Y, Makino T, et al. Single-incision laparoscopic intragastric surgery for gastric submucosal tumor located adjacent to esophagogastric junction: Report of four cases. Journal of Laparoendoscopic & Advanced Surgical Techniques. Part A. 2018;**28**(1):78-82. DOI: 10.1089/lap.2017.0026

[37] Aldrighetti L, Guzzetti E, Ferla G. Laparoscopic hepatic left lateral sectionectomy using the Laparoendoscopic Single Site approach: Evolution of minimally invasive liver surgery. Journal of Hepato-Biliary-Pancreatic Sciences. 2011;**18**:103-105. DOI: 10.1007/s00534-010-0280-6

[38] Karabicak I, Karabulut K. Single port laparoscopic liver surgery: A minireview. World Journal of Gastrointestinal Endoscopy. 2016;**8**(12):444-450. DOI: 10.4253/wjge.v8.i12.444

[39] Chatzizacharias NA, Dajani K, Koong JK, Jah A. The role of the single incision laparoscopic approach in liver and pancreatic resectional surgery. Minimally Invasive Surgery. 2016;**2016**:1454026. DOI: 10.1155/2016/1454026

[40] Pan M, Jiang Z, Cheng Y, Xu X, Zhang Z, Zhou C, et al. Single-incision laparoscopic hepatectomy for benign and malignant hepatopathy: Initial experience in 8 Chinese patients.

Surgical Innovation. 2012;**19**:446-451. DOI: 10.1177/1553350612438412

[41] Dapri G, Dimarco L, Cadi'ere GB, Donckier V. Initial experience in single-incision transumbilical laparoscopic liver resection: Indications, potential benefits, and limitations. HPB Surgery. 2012;**2012**:921973. DOI: 10.1155/2012/921973

[42] Zhao G, Hu M, Liu MR, Xu D, Ouyang C, Xu Y, et al. Laparoendoscopic single-site liver resection: A preliminary report of 12 cases. Surgical Endoscopy. 2011;**25**(10):3286-3293. DOI: 10.1007/s00464-011-1706-1

[43] Gaujoux S, Kingham TP, Jarnagin WR, D'Angelica MI, Allen PJ, Fong Y. Single-incision laparoscopic liver resection. Surgical Endoscopy. 2011;**25**:1489-1494. DOI: 10.1007/s00464-010-1419-x

[44] Shetty GS, You YK, Choi HJ, Na GH, Hong TH, Kim DG. Extending the limitations of liver surgery: Outcomes of initial human experience in a high-volume centre performing single-port laparoscopic liver resection for hepatocellular carcinoma. Surgical Endoscopy. 2012;**26**:1602-1608. DOI: 10.1007/s00464-011-2077-3

[45] Weiss M, Mittermair C, Brunner E, Schirnhofer J, Obrist C, Pimpl K, et al. Inline radiofrequency pre-coagulation simplifies single-incision laparoscopic minor liver resection. Journal of Hepato-Biliary-Pancreatic Sciences. 2015;**22**:831-836. DOI: 10.1002/jhbp.295

[46] Benzing C, Krenzien F, Atanasov G, Seehofer D, Sucher R, Zorron R, et al. Single incision laparoscopic liver resection (SILL)—A systematic review. GMS Interdisciplinary Plastic and Reconstructive Surgery DGPW. 2015;**4**:Doc17. DOI: 10.3205/iprs000076

[47] Hu M, Zhao G, Wang F, Xu D, Liu R. Single-port and multi-port laparoscopic left lateral liver sectionectomy for treating benign liver diseases: A prospective, randomized, controlled study. World Journal of Surgery. 2014;**38**:2668-2673. DOI: 10.1007/s00268-014-2610-3

[48] Aldrighetti L, Ratti F, Catena M, Pulitanò C, Ferla F, Cipriani F, et al. Laparoendoscopic single site (LESS) surgery for left-lateral hepatic sectionectomy as an alternative to traditional laparoscopy: Case-matched analysis from a single center. Surgical Endoscopy. 2012;**26**:2016-2022. DOI: 10.1007/s00464-012-2147-1

[49] Struecker B, Haber P, Öllinger R, Bahra M, Pascher A, Pratschke J, et al. Comparison of single-port versus standard multiport left lateral liver sectionectomy. Surgical Innovation. 2018;**25**(2):136-141. DOI: 10.1177/1553350617752010

[50] Choi HJ, You YK, Na GH, Hong TH, Shetty GS, Kim DG. Single-port laparoscopy-assisted donor right hepatectomy in living donor liver transplantation: Sensible approach or unnecessary hindrance? Transplantation Proceedings. 2012;**44**(2):347-352. DOI: 10.1016/j.transproceed.2012.01.018

[51] Han JH, You YK, Choi HJ, Hong TH, Kim DG. Clinical advantages of single port laparoscopic hepatectomy. World Journal of Gastroenterology. 2018;**24**(3):379-386. DOI: 10.3748/wjg.v24.i3.379

[52] Chuang SH, Lin CS. Single-incision laparoscopic surgery for biliary tract disease. World Journal of Gastroenterology. 2016;**22**(2):736-747. DOI: 10.3748/wjg.v22.i2.736

[53] Yamazaki M, Yasuda H, Koda K. Single-incision laparoscopic cholecystectomy: A systematic review of methodology and outcomes. Surgery Today. 2015;**45**(5):537-548. DOI: 10.1007/s00595-014-0908-2

[54] Schlager A, Khalaileh A, Shussman N, Elazary R, Keidar A, Pikarsky AJ, et al. Providing more through less: Current methods of retraction in SIMIS and NOTES cholecystectomy. Surgical Endoscopy. 2010;**24**(7):1542-1546. DOI: 10.1007/s00464-009-0807-6

[55] Markar SR, Karthikesalingam A, Thrumurthy S, Muirhead L, Kinross J, Paraskeva P. Single-incision laparoscopic surgery (SILS) vs. conventional multiport cholecystectomy: Systematic review and meta-analysis. Surgical Endoscopy. 2012;**26**(5):1205-1213. DOI: 10.1007/s00464-011-2051-0

[56] Garg P, Thakur JD, Garg M, Menon GR. Single-incision laparoscopic cholecystectomy vs. conventional laparoscopic cholecystectomy: A meta-analysis of randomized controlled trials. Journal of Gastrointestinal Surgery. 2012;**16**(8):1618-1628. DOI: 10.1007/s11605-012-1906-6

[57] Pisanu A, Reccia I, Porceddu G, Uccheddu A. Meta-analysis of prospective randomized studies comparing single-incision laparoscopic cholecystectomy (SILC) and conventional multiport laparoscopic cholecystectomy (CMLC). Journal of Gastrointestinal Surgery. 2012;**16**(9):1790-1801. DOI: 10.1007/s11605-012-1956-9

[58] Trastulli S, Cirocchi R, Desiderio J, Guarino S, Santoro A, Parisi A, et al. Systematic review and meta-analysis of randomized clinical trials comparing single-incision versus conventional laparoscopic cholecystectomy. The British Journal of Surgery. 2013;**100**(2):191-208. DOI: 10.1002/bjs.8937

[59] Hao L, Liu M, Zhu H, Li Z. Single-incision versus conventional laparoscopic cholecystectomy in patients with uncomplicated gallbladder disease: A meta-analysis. Surgical Laparoscopy, Endoscopy & Percutaneous Techniques. 2012;**22**(6):487-497. DOI: 10.1097/SLE.0b013e3182685d0a

[60] Wu XS, Shi LB, Gu J, Dong P, Lu JH, Li ML, et al. Single-incision laparoscopic cholecystectomy versus multi-incision laparoscopic cholecystectomy: A meta-analysis of randomized clinical trials. Journal of Laparoendoscopic & Advanced Surgical Techniques. Part A. 2013;**23**(3):183-191. DOI: 10.1089/lap.2012.0189

[61] Milas M, Deveđija S, Trkulja V. Single incision versus standard multiport laparoscopic cholecystectomy: Up-dated systematic review and meta-analysis of randomized trials. The Surgeon. 2014;**12**(5):271-289. DOI: 10.1016/j.surge.2014.01.009

[62] Geng L, Sun C, Bai J. Single incision versus conventional laparoscopic cholecystectomy outcomes: A meta-analysis of randomized controlled trials. PLoS One. 2013;**8**(10):e76530. DOI: 10.1371/journal.pone.0076530

[63] Zehetner J, Pelipad D, Darehzereshki A, Mason RJ, Lipham JC, Katkhouda N. Single-access laparoscopic cholecystectomy versus classic laparoscopic cholecystectomy: A systematic review and meta-analysis of randomized controlled trials. Surgical Laparoscopy, Endoscopy & Percutaneous Techniques. 2013;**23**(3):235-243. DOI: 10.1097/SLE.0b013e31828b8b4e

[64] Evers L, Bouvy N, Branje D, Peeters A. Single-incision laparoscopic cholecystectomy versus conventional four-port laparoscopic cholecystectomy: A systematic review and meta-analysis. Surgical Endoscopy. 2017;**31**(9):3437-3448. DOI: 10.1007/s00464-016-5381-0

[65] Haueter R, Schütz T, Raptis DA, Clavien PA, Zuber M. Meta-analysis of single-port versus conventional laparoscopic cholecystectomy

comparing body image and cosmesis. The British Journal of Surgery. 2017;**104**(9):1141-1159. DOI: 10.1002/bjs.10574

[66] Arezzo A, Passera R, Forcignanò E, Rapetti L, Cirocchi R, Morino M. Single-incision laparoscopic cholecystectomy is responsible for increased adverse events: Results of a meta-analysis of randomized controlled trials. Surgical Endoscopy. 2018;**32**(9):3739-3753. DOI: 10.1007/s00464-018-6143-y

[67] Hey J, Roberts KJ, Morris-Stiff GJ, Toogood GJ. Patient views through the keyhole: New perspectives on single-incision vs. multiport laparoscopic cholecystectomy. HPB: The Official Journal of the International Hepato Pancreato Biliary Association. 2012;**14**(4):242-246. DOI: 10.1111/j.1477-2574.2011.00435.x

[68] Yeo D, Mackay S, Martin D. Single-incision laparoscopic cholecystectomy with routine intraoperative cholangiography and common bile duct exploration via the umbilical port. Surgical Endoscopy. 2012;**26**:1122-1127. DOI: 10.1007/s00464-011-2009-2

[69] Shibao K, Higure A, Yamaguchi K. Laparoendoscopic single-site common bile duct exploration using the manual manipulator. Surgical Endoscopy. 2013;**27**:3009-3015. DOI: 10.1007/s00464-013-2837-3

[70] Tian Y, Wu S, Chen CC, Chen Y. Laparoendoscopic single-site cholecystectomy and common bile duct exploration using conventional instruments. International Journal of Surgery. 2016;**33**:140-145. DOI: 10.1016/j.ijsu.2016.07.074

[71] Kim SJ, Kim KH, An CH, Kim JS. Innovative technique of needlescopic grasper-assisted single-incision laparoscopic common bile duct exploration: A comparative study. World Journal of Gastroenterology. 2015;**21**(45):12857-12864. DOI: 10.3748/wjg.v21.i45

[72] Chuang SH, Chen PH, Chang CM, Tsai YF, Lin CS. Single incision laparoscopic common bile duct exploration with conventional instruments: An innovative technique and a comparative study. Journal of Gastrointestinal Surgery. 2014;**18**:737-743. DOI: 10.1007/s11605-013-2420-1

[73] Chuang SH, Yeh MC, Chang CJ. Laparoscopic transfistulous bile duct exploration for Mirizzi syndrome type II: A simplified standardized technique. Surgical Endoscopy. 2016;**30**:5635-5646. DOI: 10.1007/s00464-016-4911-0

[74] Chuang SH, Hung MC, Huang SW, Chou DA, Wu HS. Single-incision laparoscopic common bile duct exploration in 101 consecutive patients: Choledochotomy, transcystic, and transfistulous approaches. Surgical Endoscopy. 2018;**32**(1):485-497. DOI: 10.1007/s00464-017-5658-y

[75] Yao D, Wu S, Li Y, Chen Y, Yu X, Han J. Transumbilical single-incision laparoscopic distal pancreatectomy: Preliminary experience and comparison to conventional multi-port laparoscopic surgery. BMC Surgery. 2014;**14**:105. DOI: 10.1186/1471-2482-14-105

[76] Maemura K, Shinchi H, Mataki Y, Kurahara H, Hayashi T, Kuwahata T, et al. Advanced staging laparoscopy using single-incision approach for unresectable pancreatic cancer. Surgical Laparoscopy, Endoscopy & Percutaneous Techniques. 2011;**21**(6):e301-e305. DOI: 10.1097/SLE.0b013e31823bae57

[77] Subramaniam D, Dunn WK, Simpson J. Novel use of a single port laparoscopic surgery device for minimally invasive pancreatic necrosectomy. Annals of the

Royal College of Surgeons of England. 2012;**94**:438. DOI: 10.1308/003588412X13373405386015a

[78] Machado MA, Surjan RC, Makdissi FF. Laparoscopic distal pancreatectomy using single-port platform: Technique, safety, and feasibility in a clinical case series. Journal of Laparoendoscopic & Advanced Surgical Techniques. Part A. 2015;**25**(7):581-585. DOI: 10.1089/lap.2015.0032

[79] Chang SK, Lomanto D, Mayasari M. Single-port laparoscopic spleen preserving distal pancreatectomy. Minimally Invasive Surgery. 2012;**2012**:197429. DOI: 10.1155/2012/197429

[80] Barbaros U, Sümer A, Demirel T, et al. Single incision laparoscopic pancreas resection for pancreatic metastasis of renal cell carcinoma. Journal of the Society of Laparoendoscopic Surgeons. 2010;**14**:566-570. DOI: 10.4293/108680810X12924466008448

[81] Misawa T, Ito R, Futagawa Y, Fujiwara Y, Kitamura H, Tsutsui N, et al. Single-incision laparoscopic distal pancreatectomy with or without splenic preservation: How we do it. Asian Journal of Endoscopic Surgery. 2012;**5**(4):195-199. DOI: 10.1111/j.1758-5910.2012.00155.x

[82] Srikanth G, Shetty N, Dubey D. Single incision laparoscopic distal pancreatectomy with splenectomy for neuroendocrine tumor of the tail of pancreas. Journal of Minimal Access Surgery. 2013;**9**(3):132-135. DOI: 10.4103/0972-9941.115377

[83] Han HJ, Yoon SY, Song TJ, Choi SB, Kim WB, Choi SY, et al. Single-port laparoscopic distal pancreatectomy: Initial experience. Journal of Laparoendoscopic & Advanced Surgical Techniques. Part A. 2014;**24**(12):858-863. DOI: 10.1089/lap.2014.0151

[84] Haugvik SP, Røsok BI, Waage A, Mathisen O, Edwin B. Single-incision versus conventional laparoscopic distal pancreatectomy: A single-institution case-control study. Langenbeck's Archives of Surgery. 2013;**398**(8):1091-1096. DOI: 10.1007/s00423-013-1133-y

[85] Han HJ, Kang CM. Reduced port minimally invasive distal pancreatectomy: Single-port laparoscopic versus robotic single-site plus one-port distal pancreatectomy. Surgical Endoscopy. 11 Jul 2018. DOI: 10.1007/s00464-018-6361-3

[86] Habermalz B, Sauerland S, Decker G, Delaitre B, Gigot JF, Leandros E, et al. Laparoscopic splenectomy: The clinical practice guidelines of the European Association for Endoscopic Surgery (EAES). Surgical Endoscopy. 2008;**242**:821-848. DOI: 10.1007/s00464-007-9735-5

[87] Barbaros U, Dinççağ A. Single incision laparoscopic splenectomy: The first two cases. Journal of Gastrointestinal Surgery. 2009;**13**:1520-1523. DOI: 10.1007/s11605-009-0869-8

[88] Fan Y, Wu SD, Kong J, Su Y, Tian Y, Yu H. Feasibility and safety of single-incision laparoscopic splenectomy: A systematic review. The Journal of Surgical Research. 2014;**186**:354-362. DOI: 10.1016/j.jss.2013.09.010

[89] Targarona EM, Lima MB, Balague C, Trias M. Single-port splenectomy: Current update and controversies. Journal of Minimal Access Surgery. 2011;**7**(1):61-64. DOI: 10.4103/0972-9941.72383

[90] Misawa T, Sakamoto T, Ito R, Shiba H, Gocho T, Wakiyama S, et al. Single-incision laparoscopic splenectomy using the "tug-exposure technique" in adults: Results of ten initial cases. Surgical Endoscopy. 2011;**25**(10):3222-3227. DOI: 10.1007/s00464-011-1697-y

[91] Monclova JL, Targarona EM, Vidal P, Peraza Y, Garcia F, Otero CR, et al. Single incision versus reduced port splenectomy—Searching for the best alternative to conventional laparoscopic splenectomy. Surgical Endoscopy. 2013;**27**(3):895-902. DOI: 10.1007/s00464-012-2530-y

[92] Wu S, Lai H, Zhao J, Deng X, Wei J, Liang J, et al. Systematic review and meta-analysis of single-incision versus conventional multiport laparoscopic splenectomy. Journal of Minimal Access Surgery. 2018;**14**(1):1-8. DOI: 10.4103/0972-9941.195573

Section 3

Endometriosis Surgery

Chapter 5

New Paradigms in Endometriosis Surgery of the Distal Ureter

José Anacleto Dutra de Resende Júnior, Rodrigo Ribeiro Vieiralves, Renata Teles Buere and Claudio Peixoto Crispi

Abstract

It is estimated that 2% of endometriosis cases involve the urinary tract and that the ureter is involved in up to 30% of these cases, or 0.6% of all endometriosis cases. Increasingly, the standardization and systematization of surgical treatment of endometriosis require the surgeon to have knowledge of the surgical spaces and the ureteral and surrounding pelvic anatomy in order to carry out a cytoreductive surgery that is as possible. A thorough workup is essential for the differentiation of intrinsic or extrinsic endometriosis of the ureter. The use of the resonance imaging preoperatively and ureteroscopy intraoperatively is now considered indispensable. The decision and choice of the best technique will be guided by the diagnosis (intrinsic or extrinsic), the location of the lesions, the length of the involved segment (greater or less than 3 cm), vitality of the ureter stumps, and anastomosis without tension. The main alternatives are ureterolysis and dilatation with balloon catheter which is performed for extrinsic endometriosis more than 85% of the time and ureterectomy for intrinsic endometriosis. To perform the reconstruction, the techniques with end-to-end anastomosis with the distal ureter stump or uretero-vesical reimplantation are used. Increasingly, with better knowledge of the distal ureter anatomy, easier access through laparoscopy and in contradiction to the current recommendations, we are verifying that the end-to-end anastomosis has become the preferred option *or* procedure of choice for ureteral reconstruction, with ureterovesical reimplantation the second option.

Keywords: endometriosis, ureter, laparoscopic surgery, new technique, new surgical approach

1. Introduction

Endometriosis involving the urinary tract is rare, affecting only 1–2% of women with endometriosis. The vast majority of these cases – 80–85% involve the bladder. Ureteral endometriosis occurs in just 15% of cases. Ureteral involvement usually occurs near its insertion in the bladder, just above the ureterovesical junction (UVJ), near where it crosses the uterine artery [1–6]. We believe that this prevalence is underestimated due to the scarce data in the literature and the lack of standardization of the surgical technique around the world in different countries. Based on our practical experience, we believe that extrinsic ureter involvement is more prevalent than the data in the literature would suggest, and may exceed 30% of all surgeries for multicompartmental deep endometriosis, especially when there is intestinal (rectal/sigmoid) infiltration and/or parametrical infiltration. Thus, knowledge of ureteral endometriosis and its management are of fundamental importance for surgeons who propose to perform comprehensive treatment of the various presentations of endometriosis.

2. Ureter anatomy

The ureter connects the renal pelvis to the bladder, typically measuring 20–30 cm in length. It is a tubular conduit with a smooth muscle structure that confers a capacity for peristalsis. The ureter's course is entirely retroperitoneal; for didactic purposes it is divided into two portions: abdominal and pelvic. The abdominal portion maintains an important relation with the psoas muscle and gonadal vessels, traveling laterally to the latter throughout its abdominal course. Before penetrating the pelvis, uteter passes anteriorly to the iliac vessels, and the pelvic segment initially accompanies the internal iliac artery (**Figure 1**).

In the female, the pelvic segment of the ureter penetrates the parametrium and courses between the uterine artery (above) and vaginal artery (below). At this

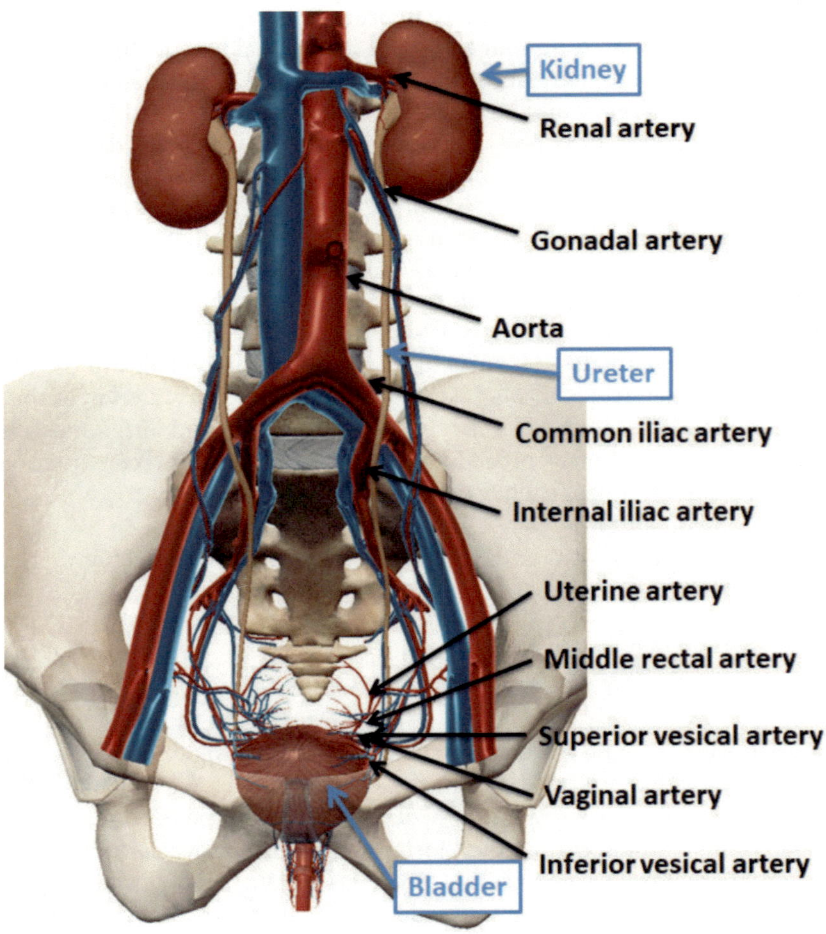

Figure 1.
Vascular supply of the uterers and their relation to the great vessels.

point, great care must be taken in its identification, as iatrogenic injuries of the ureter may occur during pelvic surgeries.

The ureter is irrigated by multiple arteries along its course, starting with the renal, gonadal, aorta and common iliac arteries. More distally in its pelvic segment the ureter is supplied by the internal iliac, superior vesicle, uterine, medial rectal arteries, vaginal, and inferior vesicle arteries (**Figure 1**). As they approach the ureter, the arterial branches travel along a longitudinal pathway within the adventitia (ureteral sheath), forming anastomotic bundles. In this way the surgical dissection of the ureter should strive to preserve the adventitia in order to avoid ischemia.

3. Classification: extrinsic versus intrinsic

Endometriosis can infiltrate the ureter intrinsically or extrinsically. When extrinsic – 80–90% of such cases – the endometriosis infiltrates the adventitia and/or submucosa. When intrinsic (the remainder of cases), the disease infiltrates the mucosa and submucosa and may present as ureteral stenosis [5, 7].

4. Clinical and imaging work-up

A thorough history and physical examination are essential in order to recognize or suspect urological impairment secondary to endometriosis. The patient may be asymptomatic or experience cyclical renal colic and hematuria during the menstrual period. In intrinsic cases the endometriosis may progress to obstruct the lumen of the ureter, whereas in extrinsic cases there can be circumferential or annular (extrinsic) compression. Both are capable of insidiously causing partial and even complete loss of renal function in one or both kidneys.

Assessment using imaging studies is indispensable for surgical planning. Not all anatomical sites are accessible to ultrasound. Magnetic resonance imaging can identify and assess hemorrhagic components of endometriomas throughout the pelvis, and thus is the preferred imaging method to assess ureteral involvement (**Figure 2**).

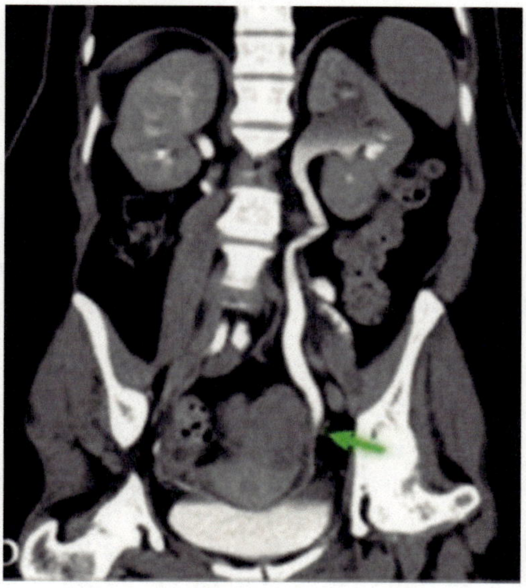

Figure 2.
Endometriosis infiltrating the left ureter (green arrow) generating ureterohydronephrosis.

In cases in which impaired renal function is known or suspected, static and dynamic renal scintigraphy should be ordered, and endoscopic investigation (ureteroscopy) contemplated to inform surgical planning.

Preoperative cystoscopy to evaluate bladder endometriosis is necessary especially when a non-invasive imaging method (MRI or ultrasonography) identifies lesions which are suspicious for endometriosis in the compartment anterior to the uterus. In the cases of lesions infiltrating the bladder mucosa, it is important to determine the exact location(s), their size and their distance from the two ureteral ostia, as well as any projection into the ureter intramurally.

Such findings could help determine which surgical approach should be used; options range from simple ureterolysis to ureterectomy with uretero-ureteral anastomosis or a ureterovesical reimplantation. Concomitant cystoscopy with vaginal palpation is important to assess disease or areas of adhesions localized in the vesicouterine septum that may suggest the need for partial cystectomy or suture-reinforced bladder shaving (**Figure 3**).

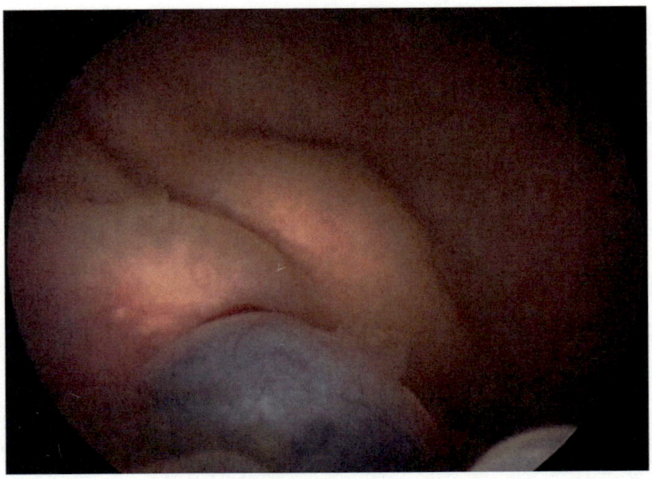

Figure 3.
Endometriosis infiltrating the bladder trigone and right ureteral ostium as visualized during cystoscopy.

5. Preoperative preparation

It is advisable to perform outpatient urinary sediment (EAS) and urine culture studies preoperatively to ensure sterile urine during the procedure.

Antimicrobial prophylaxis should be administrated during the induction of anesthesia. Thromboembolic prophylaxis of the lower extremities with compressive or pneumatic stockings is also recommended.

6. Surgical treatment

Treatment of endometriosis should be individualized. The laparoscopic approach, robot-assisted or not, has become the option o choice for most surgeons [8, 9]. We observed that through accumulated experience and continuous training, it becomes possible to carry out increasingly complex cases laparoscopically, affording the patient all the advantages and benefits of minimally invasive techniques.

6.1 Laparoscopic tools and materials used

The basic laparoscopic surgical tools required include non-traumatic grasping forceps, Maryland forceps, laparoscopic scissors, laparoscopic needle holders and contra-need holders, as well as an articulating Hook with monopolar cautery. No special clamps are required for this procedure. Bipolar or ultrasonic clamps when available will help with the dissection and hemostasis, reducing surgical time.

Contemplating the possibility of a joint intervention – laparoscopy and cystoscopy/ureteroscopy – a cystoscope, ureteroscope, hydrophilic guidewire, and ureteral catheter should be available. If there is more intense manipulation or segmental resection of the ureter, double J catheter placement will be necessary, in order to ensure a patent ureter and adequate healing. It is worth mentioning that inoperative dynamic C-arm fluoroscopy should be available to verify proper positioning of the catheters.

6.2 Positioning the patient

How the patient is positioned for surgery will depend on the site of ureteral involvement. For the more common case of distal involvement, the patient should be placed in the Lloyd Davies and Trendelenburg position, lying directly on a non-adherent eggcrate foam pad. The legs should be wrapped in pneumatic stockings and secured to boot-like leggings, avoiding continuous compression of the calves.

6.3 Surgical approach: Access

The first puncture is performed in the umbilical scar where a 10 mm trocar is placed to introduce the optic (**Figure 4**–black circle) and the patient is kept in dorsal decubitus. After exploration of the cavity, the patient is placed in Trendelenburg (Lloyd Davies) position and the surgeon inserts two 5 mm trocars (**Figure 4**–blue circles) and a fourth trocar for the first assistant. The second assistant stands between the patient's legs to manipulate the uterus after placement of the uterine manipulator (**Figure 4**–second assistant). With the surgical team members in these positions it is possible to perform ureterolysis, uretero-ureteral anastomosis and ureterovesical reimplantations on the right (**Figure 4-A**) or on the left (**Figure 4-B**).

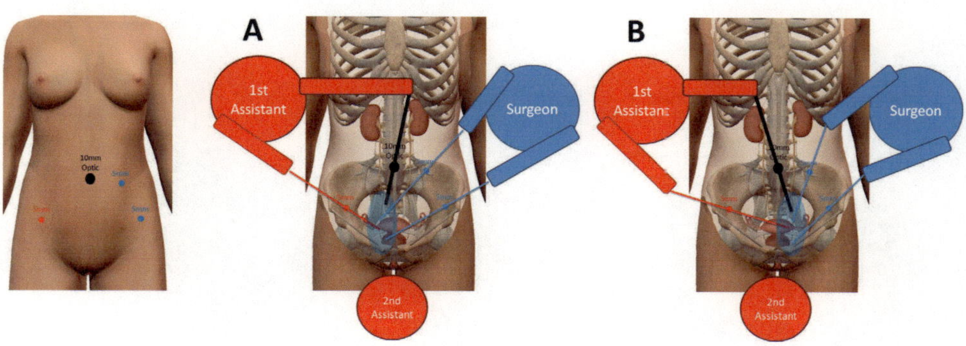

Figure 4.
Trocar sites. Position of surgeons for access to the right distal ureter (A) and for access to the left distal ureter (B).

6.4 Surgical approach–ureterolysis, ureterectomy and end-to-end anastomosis or ureteral replantation

In endometriosis that involves the ureter, we may encounter ureteral involvement due to fibrosis without extrinsic muscle/muscular infiltration or intrinsic endometriosis infiltrating the muscular layer and/or mucosa. It is only after ureterolysis of the entire affected section of the ureter and segments proximal and distal portions to the disease that the surgical approach can be assessed/determined (**Figure 5**) and (**Figures 10–12**). It is always important to perform a ureteroscopy (**Figures 6** and **13**) to evaluate the internal aspect/lumen of this ureter and if necessary to perform a frozen biopsy to confirm or rule out the possibility of intrinsic endometriosis.

With extrinsic disease – the majority of cases – with careful ureterolysis using "cold" scissors all disease can be removed without the need to resect any segment of the ureter (**Figures 7** and **8**). After a laborious ureterolysis, it is recommended that the narrowed segment be dilated using a ureteral balloon catheter dilator (**Figure 9**) endoscopically either by cystoscopy or ureteroscopy, with placement of a double J catheter for 30–60 days.

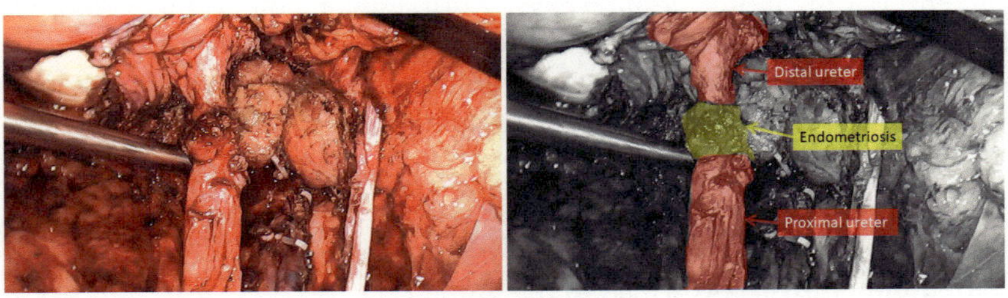

Figure 5.
Ureterolysis with identification of segments proximal and distal to the endometriosis.

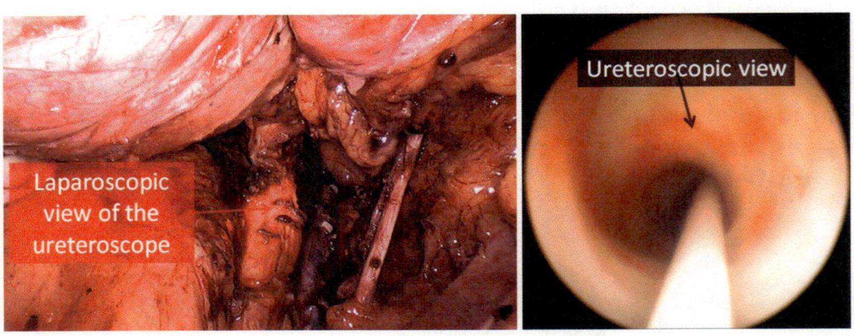

Figure 6.
Laparoscopic and ureteroscopic views of the ureteral segment with extrinsic endometriosis.

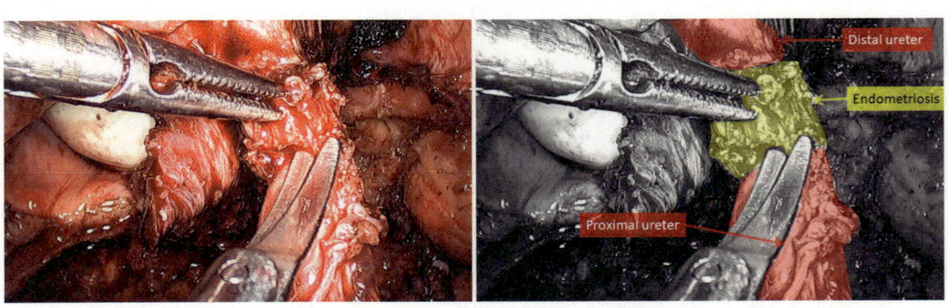

Figure 7.
Dissection of the ureter using scissors (without energy) - initiation of the freeing of the extrinsic endometriosis.

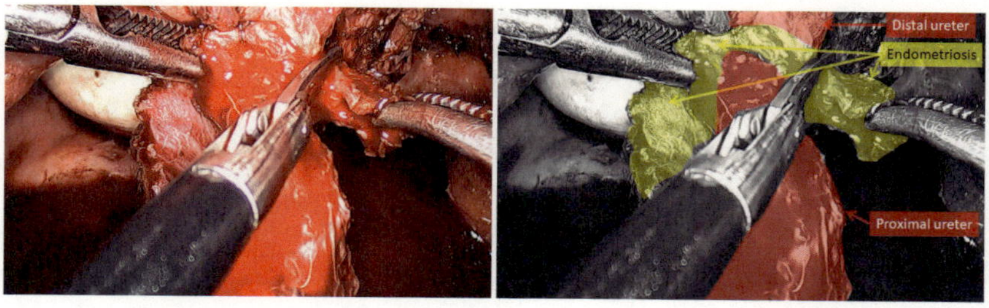

Figure 8.
Dissection of the ureter with freeing of the extrinsic endometriosis.

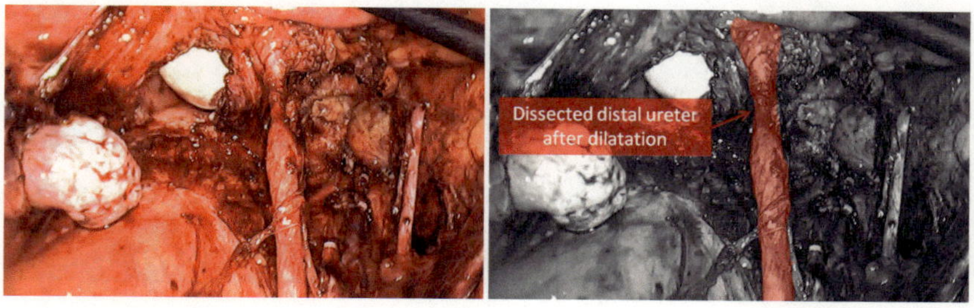

Figure 9.
Dilatation of the stented segment using a balloon catheter (laparoscopic view) and posterior placement of the double J catheter.

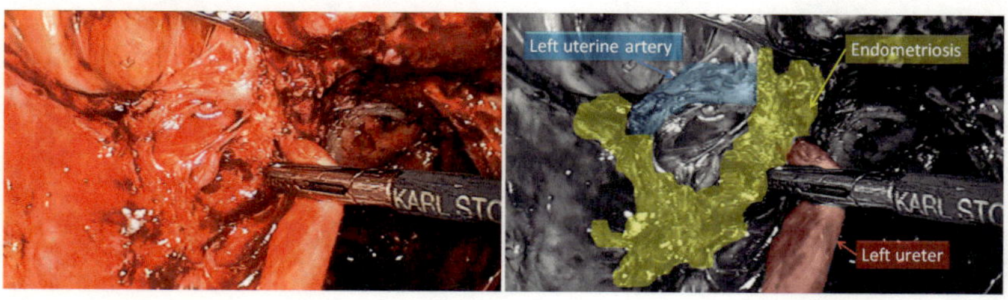

Figure 10.
Left parametric endometriosis involving the ureter at the intersection of the uterine artery.

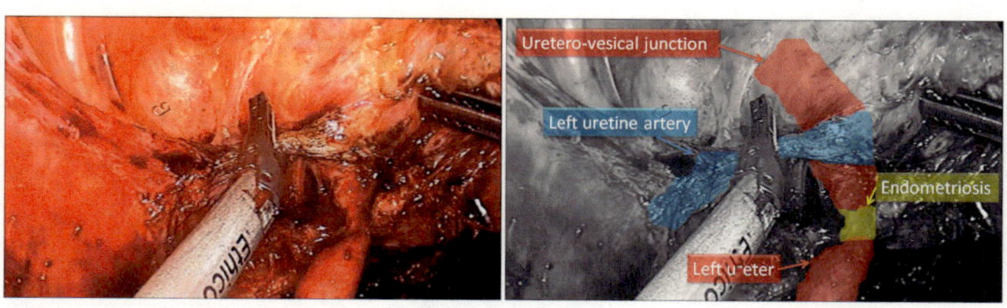

Figure 11.
Ligature of the uterine artery to access the distal ureter and identification of the uretero-vesical junction (UVJ).

When ureteroscopy reveals intrinsic endometriosis (**Figure 13**), (typically 3–4 cm from the UVJ) ureterectomy of the involved segment is necessary (**Figures 10–16**) subject to consideration of the best surgical technique [10]. In those cases where the distal ureter stump (close to the UVJ) is greater than 1 cm, one can elect to perform an end-to-end ureteroureterostomy (**Figure 17**), another ureteroscopy after the anastomosis (**Figure 18**), with placement of a double J catheter [11, 12].

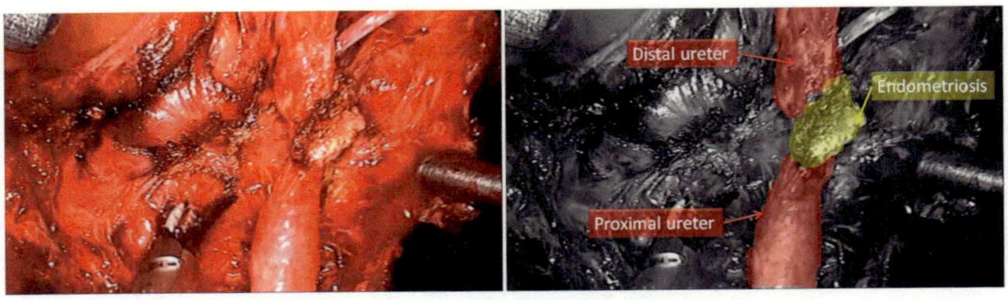

Figure 12.
Ureterolysis with identification of segments proximal and distal to the endometriosis.

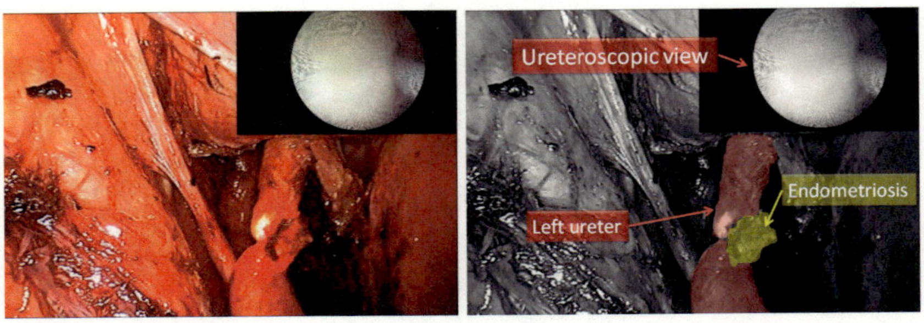

Figure 13.
Ureteroscopy with identification of the intrinsic lesion and obstruction to the passage of the ureteroscope.

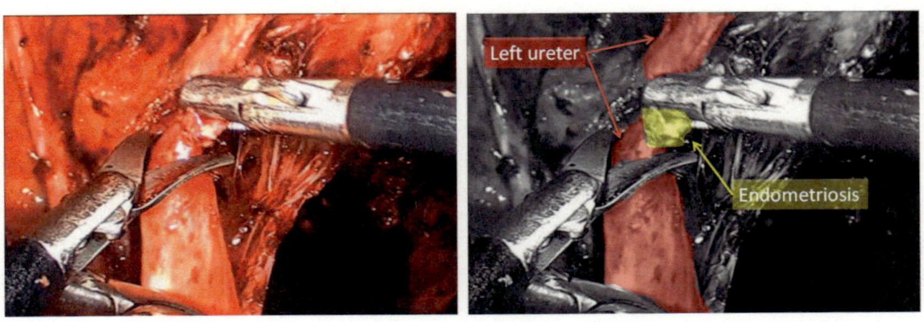

Figure 14.
Proximal ureterectomy. Section with spatulation of the ureter proximal to the lesion.

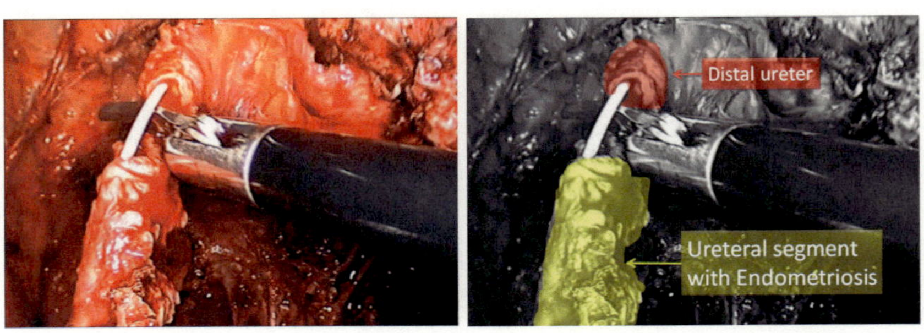

Figure 15.
Distal ureterectomy. Section with spreading of the ureter distal to the lesion and separation of the segment with endometriosis.

In cases in which the distal ureteral stump is very small (less than 1 cm) or the endometriotic lesion infiltrates the ureter intramurally and the bladder (via the ureteral ostium), a uretero-vesical reimplantation is required [13, 14] (**Figures 19–26**).

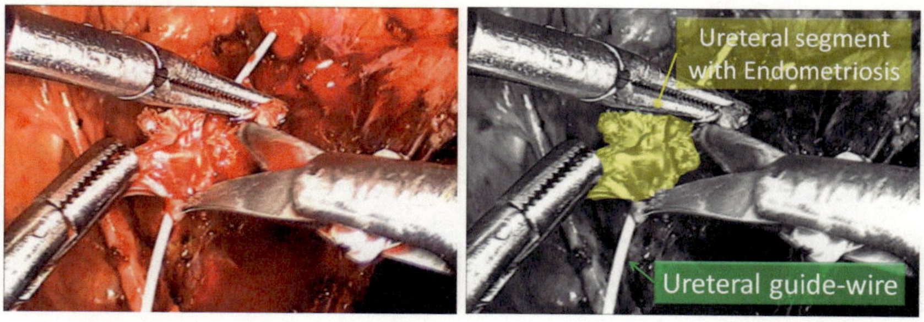

Figure 16.
Section and removal of the segment with endometriosis on the ureteral guidewire.

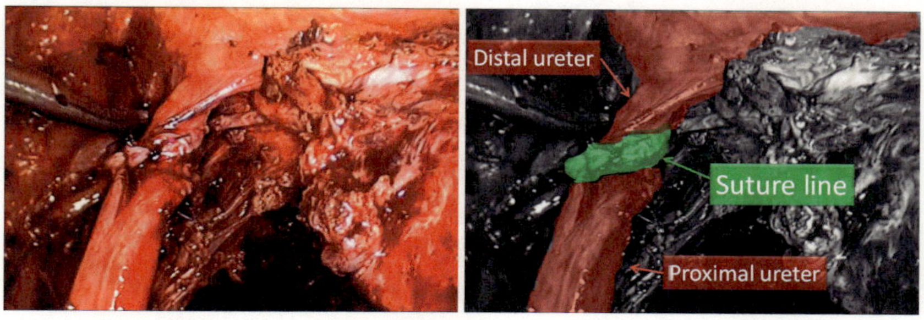

Figure 17.
Uretero-ureteral anastomosis.

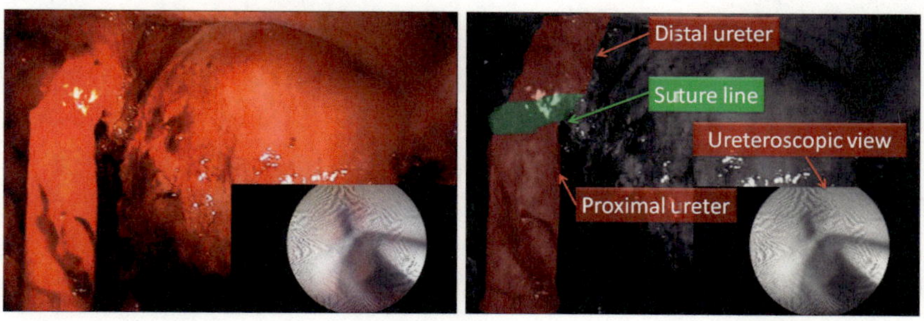

Figure 18.
Ureteroscopy of the suture line of the uretero-ureteral anastomosis.

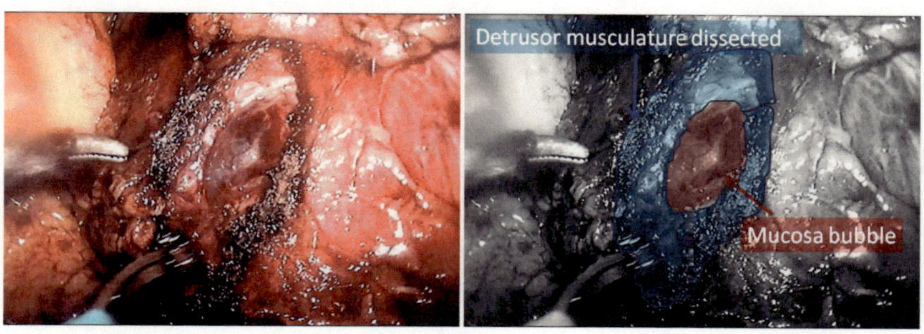

Figure 19.
Dissection of the detrusor muscles and confection of the mucosal blister.

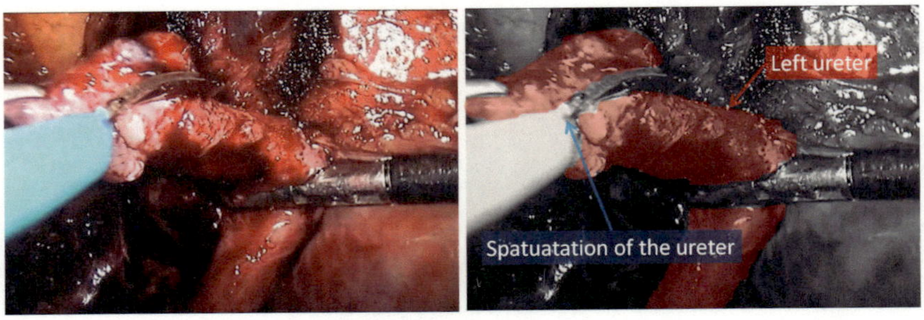

Figure 20.
Spatulation of the ureter to be implanted.

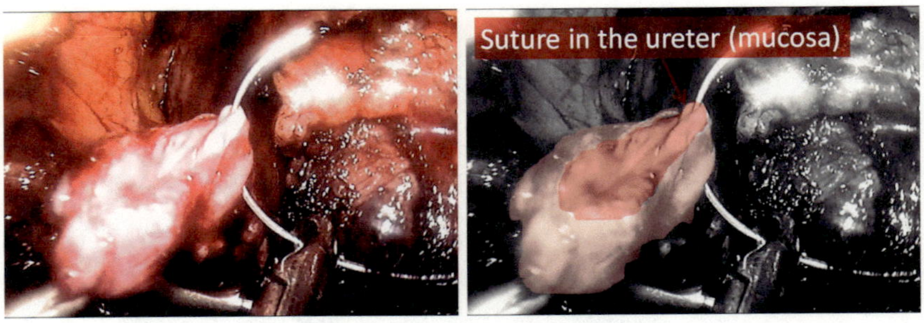

Figure 21.
Starting the anastomosis: Suture in the ureter.

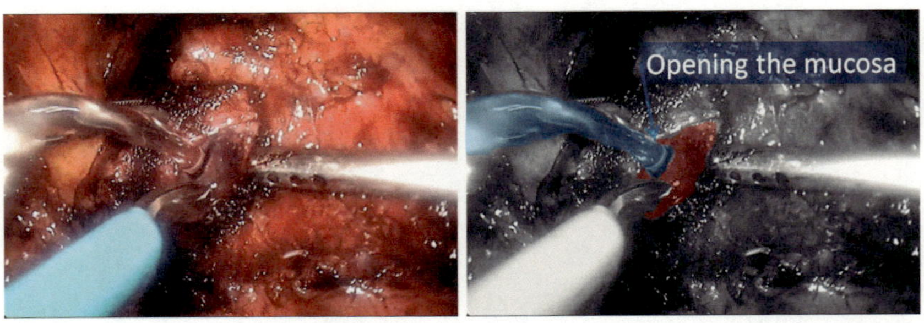

Figure 22.
Opening the bladder mucosa.

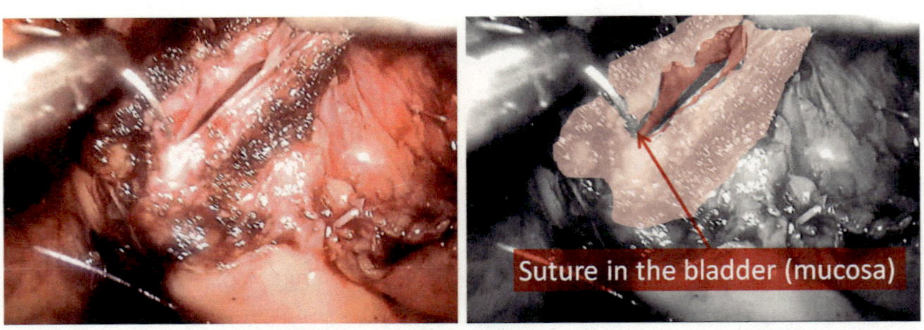

Figure 23.
First suture of the bladder anastomosis.

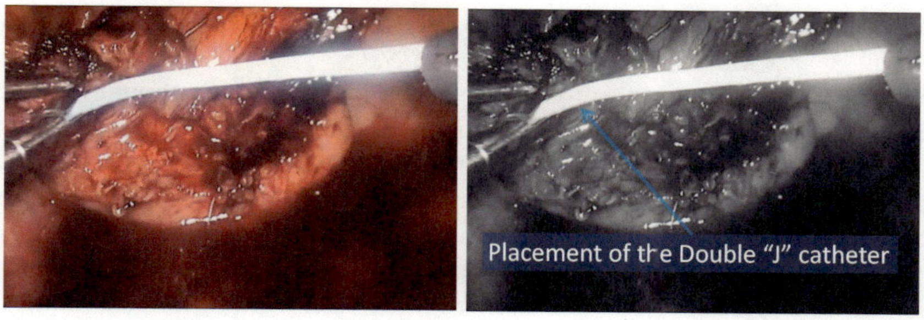

Figure 24.
Placement of the double "J" catheter.

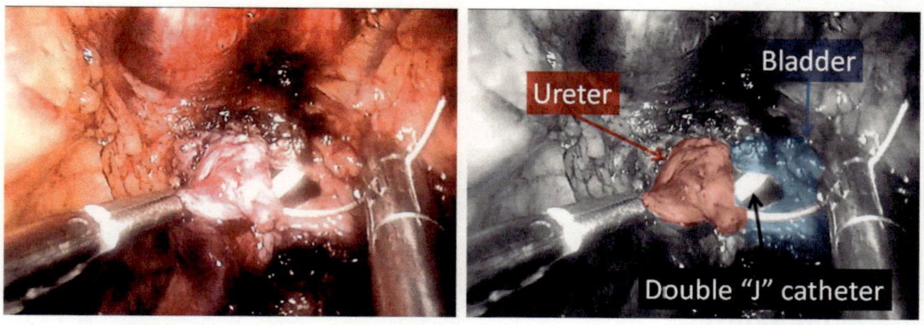

Figure 25.
End of uretero-vesical anastomosis.

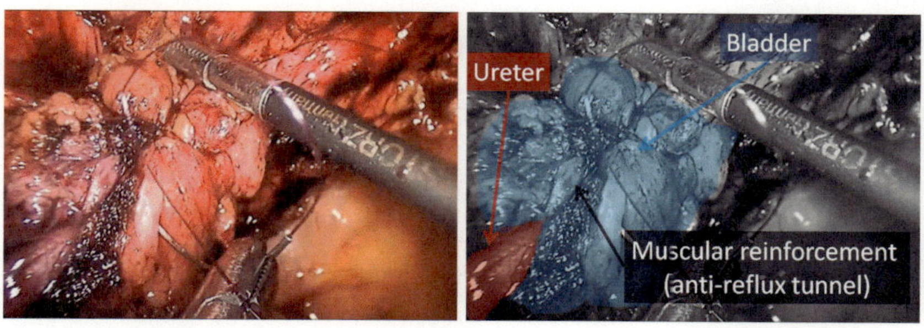

Figure 26.
Reinforcement suture of the detrusor muscles on the uretero-vesical anastomosis and on the distal ureter (anti-reflux tunnel).

7. Post-operative care

As with all transperitoneal surgery, a period of adynamic ileus should be respected after the procedure. The progression of the diet should be individualized, but typically requires less than 8 hours. Early ambulation is essential in this context, and it also helps to minimize thromboembolic events. Early administration of enoxaparin (starting 12 hours after the end of surgery) is indicated unless there are contraindications. Antibiotic prophylaxis should be restricted to the intraoperative period and certainly should not be initiated more than 24 hours after the procedure [15].

8. Complications

Given an experienced multidisciplinary team, complications should be proportional to the extent of the lesion(s). Specifically regarding ureteral endometriosis, in cases where there is a need for extensive ureterolysis, ureteral ischemia and urinary fistulas with the formation of urinomas can be observed. In cases of ureteral resection and anastomoses (uretero-ureteral anastomosis or ureteral reimplantation) anastomotic dehiscence may occur with formation of urinary fistulas. However, double J catheter placement dramatically reduces such complications. Another common complication is stenosis at the anastomosis site [9, 11, 14].

9. Conclusion

The laparoscopic surgical treatment of ureteral endometriosis is feasible provided the surgeon is trained in laparoscopic surgery and has knowledge of the ureteral anatomy and its anatomical relationships. These conditions being met, laparoscopic surgical treatment of ureteral endometriosis can be considered safe, with low rates of postoperative complications and low morbidity.

Acknowledgements

Our special thanks to Dr. Leigh J. Passman for reviewing the English manuscript.

Conflict of interest

None.

Author details

José Anacleto Dutra de Resende Júnior[1,2,3,4]*, Rodrigo Ribeiro Vieiralves[1,3,4], Renata Teles Buere[2] and Claudio Peixoto Crispi[3,4]

1 Federal Hospital of Lagoa (HFL), Rio de Janeiro, Brazil

2 Rio de Janeiro State University (UERJ), Rio de Janeiro, Brazil

3 Minimally Invasive Surgery Training Complex, Crispi Institute, Rio de Janeiro, Brazil

4 SUPREMA–Faculty of Medical Sciences and Health, Juiz de Fora, MG, Brazil

*Address all correspondence to: joseanacletojunior@gmail.com

References

[1] Vercellini P, Pisacreta A, Pesole A, Vicentini S, Stellato G, Crosignani PG. Is ureteral endometriosis an asymmetric disease? BJOG: An International Journal of Obstetrics & Gynaecology. 2000 Apr; **107**(4):559-561

[2] Resende Júnior JAD, Buere RT, Guerra CS, Sessa FV, Aragão LC, Raymundo TS, et al. Prevalence of Pre-operative Urodynamic Abnormalities in Women with DEEP Infiltrating Endometriosis: A Descriptive Study. [cited 2015 Dec 10]. Available from: http://www.ics.org/Abstracts/Publish/218/000602_poster.pdf

[3] Resende Júnior JAD, Buere RT, Guerra CGS, Raymundo TS. Urinary Symptoms and Urodynamic Findings in Women with Parametrial Endometriosis: An Exploratory StudY. [cited 2017 Jan 4]. Available from: https://www.ics.org/Abstracts/Publish/218/000608_poster.pdf

[4] Resende Júnior JAD, Buere RT, Guerra CS, Sessa FV, Raymundo TS, Oliveira MAP, et al. Dysfunctional Voiding and Urodynamic Changes in Women with Bladder Endometriosis. [cited 2015 Dec 10]. Available from: http://www.ics.org/Abstracts/Publish/218/000613_poster.pdf

[5] Donnez J, Nisolle M, Squifflet J. Ureteral endometriosis: A complication of rectovaginal endometriotic (adenomyotic) nodules. Fertility and Sterility. 2002 Jan;**77**(1):32-37

[6] Seracchioli R, Raimondo D, Di Donato N, Leonardi D, Spagnolo E, Paradisi R, et al. Histological evaluation of ureteral involvement in women with deep infiltrating endometriosis: Analysis of a large series. Human Reproduction, Oxford England. 2015 Apr;**30**(4):833-839

[7] Yohannes P. Ureteral endometriosis. The Journal of Urology. 2003 Jul;**170**(1): 20-25

[8] Hanssens S, Nisolle M, Leguevaque P, Neme RM, Cela V, Barton-Smith P, et al. Robotic-assisted laparoscopy for deep infiltrating endometriosis: The register of the Society of European Robotic Gynaecological Surgery. Gynécologie, Obstétrique & Fertilité. 2014 Nov;**42**(11):744-748

[9] Uccella S, Cromi A, Casarin J, Bogani G, Pinelli C, Serati M, et al. Laparoscopy for ureteral endometriosis: Surgical details, long-term follow-up, and fertility outcomes. Fertility and Sterility. 2014 Jul;**102**(1):160-166.e2

[10] Pérez-Utrilla Pérez M, Aguilera Bazán A, Alonso Dorrego JM, Hernández A, de Francisco MG, Martín Hernández M, et al. Urinary tract endometriosis: Clinical, diagnostic, and therapeutic aspects. Urology. 2009 Jan; **73**(1):47-51

[11] Lee Z, Llukani E, Reilly CE, Mydlo JH, Lee DI, Eun DD. Single surgeon experience with robot-assisted ureteroureterostomy for pathologies at the proximal, middle, and distal ureter in adults. Journal of Endourology. 2013 Aug;**27**(8):994-999

[12] Musch M, Hohenhorst L, Pailliart A, Loewen H, Davoudi Y, Kroepfl D. Robot-assisted reconstructive surgery of the distal ureter: Single institution experience in 16 patients. BJU International. 2013 May;**111**(5):773-783

[13] Lusuardi L, Hager M, Sieberer M, Schätz T, Kloss B, Hruby S, et al. Laparoscopic treatment of intrinsic endometriosis of the urinary tract and proposal of a treatment scheme for ureteral endometriosis. Urology. 2012 Nov;**80**(5):1033-1038

[14] Schonman R, Dotan Z, Weintraub AY, Goldenberg M, Seidman DS, Schiff E, et al. Long-term follow-up after ureteral reimplantation in patients with

severe deep infiltrating endometriosis. European Journal of Obstetrics, Gynecology, and Reproductive Biology. 2013 Nov;**171**(1):146-149

[15] Melnyk M, Casey RG, Black P, Koupparis AJ. Enhanced recovery after surgery (ERAS) protocols: Time to change practice? Canadian Urological Association Journal. 2011 Oct;**5**(5): 342-348

Section 4

Robotic Surgery

Chapter 6

Intelligent Information-Guided Robotic Surgery

Ryu Nakadate and Makoto Hashizume

Abstract

Laparoscopic surgery is minimally invasive, providing various benefits for patients. On the other hand, it is technically demanding for physicians due to limited dexterity of tools, limited vision. In order to cope with those limitations, recent various engineering technologies are trying to help surgeon. Robotics is one of the major technologies in this field. Until today, da Vinci has been only one such robot. But recently, many other robotic systems are under development. Those new robots are introduced in this chapter first. Other than robotics, or in conjunction with robotics, navigation technologies are getting popularity in clinical use. Navigation is a technology that provides useful information such as preoperative images or distance between tool and lesion, etc. to surgeon. Our experience in clinical use of navigation system in robotic surgery is introduced. Finally, technologies applied for the training of surgeon are introduced and described.

Keywords: robotic surgery, navigation surgery, computer-aided surgery, surgical training, endoscope

1. Introduction

In order to access the lesion, large incision on the healthy part of the patient, such as body surface is inevitable in the conventional (so-called open surgery) surgery. One of the modalities of the surgery which tries to minimize the incision on the healthy organ is laparoscopic surgery. The access to the lesion in the abdominal cavity is through several small incisions which sizes are about 5–10 mm. A long, slim camera and surgical devices are inserted from those incisions to the abdominal cavity. The surgeons perform surgical procedures such as incision, dissection, and suturing by manipulating those surgical devices watching a display of camera image. Compared with the conventional open surgery in which the large incision on the patient skin is made, the laparoscopic surgery provides the patients less postoperative pain and shorter hospital stay, which are the major benefits to the patients. On the other hand, the laparoscopic surgery demands high level technical skills of the surgeons because of several reasons. The surgeons lose direct vision, and only two-dimensional indirect vision through the display is available [1]. The indirect vision sometimes takes the sense of orientation and ability of the depth perception away from surgeons. All surgical devices are slim and long. The precise manipulation of the tip of those devices is very difficult. Also the mirror effect, the phenomenon in which the device in the patient body goes opposite direction to the handle outside the body, makes those manipulations more difficult [2]. The surgeons cannot directly touch the organs in the body. Palpation or feeling the applied force is not possible. Most of the surgical

IntechOpen

devices are straight, do not have bending wrist. Those devices provide surgeon much less dexterity than the fingers and hands. In order to cope with those restrictions, long training time, experience, and practices are required for the laparoscopic surgeons. However, as those limitations are mainly technical issue, we believe the technologies can contribute to overcome those limitations. In this chapter, we introduce recent various technologies for laparoscopic surgery. First, we will overview the current worldwide surgical robotics. There is a dominant player in this field, da Vinci surgical system. However, several new robots by start-ups are in the pipeline. Then, we will introduce the robotics with the flexible endoscope as a new trend in the robotic surgery. They are also in the pipeline of the many companies, about to launch to the market. We think this field is promising as future minimally invasive surgery. After that, the technologies in the navigation and training are described.

2. Robotics for the laparoscopic surgery

In this field, the da Vinci surgical system (**Figure 1**) [3] of Intuitive Surgical, Inc. (US) has been a dominant robot since its FDA approval in 2000. As of August 1, 2018, 4666 units are installed in the world. Nearly 1 million procedures in the world are performed annually by using da Vinci [4]. Majority of da Vinci applications are urology and gynecology which are about one-third of the total procedures each [4]. Including the colorectal application in the other one-third, you can find that the da Vinci surgery is mostly used in the pelvic cavity. This is probably because pelvic cavity is narrow and deep, thus laparoscopic approach is challenging for those organs such as prostate, uterus, colon, and rectum.

Generally speaking, the robot for laparoscopic surgery provides three-dimensional vision, dexterity, and intuitiveness. In fact, three-dimensional vision is not a robot specific feature. However, it is inevitable in order to exert the robotic dexterity. To understand the dexterity, let us explain the degrees of freedom. For example, in order to perform full dexterity by a grasping device, it requires seven degrees of freedom. First, the tip of the grasper has to be reached at desired position in three-dimensional space (X-Y-Z axis). Therefore, at least three degrees of freedom are required. Then, the tip of the grasper also has to change orientation at the desired position. The orientation is defined by rotations around X, Y, Z axis. Thus, it requires another three (rotational) degrees of freedom. Last, one degree of freedom is open/close motion of the grasper. Conventional laparoscopic forceps have only five degrees of freedom (three positional, one rotational around the shaft,

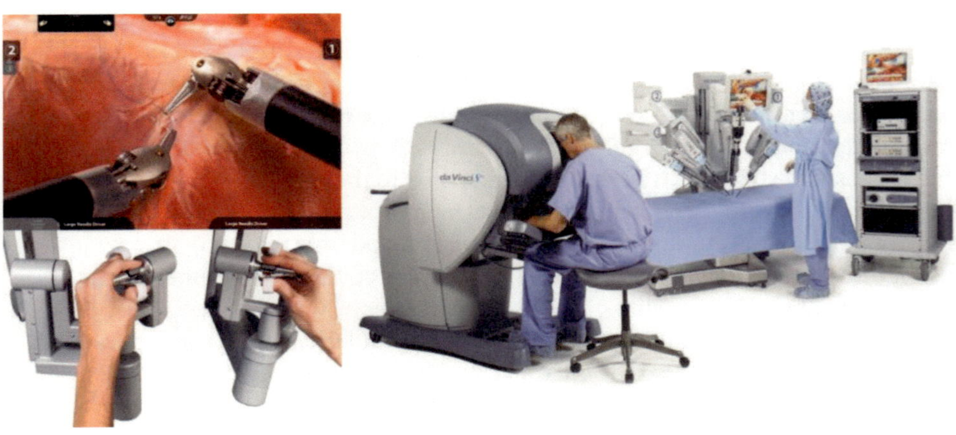

Figure 1.
da Vinci surgical system ©2018 Intuitive Surgical, Inc.

and one grasping), resulting limited dexterity. da Vinci has wrist at the tip of the forceps, providing seven degrees of freedom. This is one of the key technologies of the laparoscopic surgical robot. Intuitiveness means that the operator's hand and device tip are synchronized in the three-dimensional vision. The computer of the robot calculates the device position, so that the direction of the device movement in the display is the same as surgeon's hand. Furthermore, the computer calculation is considering the line of sight in order to secure the hand-eye coordination. Those features are basically the same in the other emerging new robots.

There exist a lot of researches on surgical robots in academic institutes. However, sometimes they are very early stage, and it is unknown how long they take time until they reach at clinically usable phase. Here, we will introduce surgical robots which have already been in the market or are in the pipeline of the industrial companies.

2.1 Senhance surgical platform

Senhance surgical robotic system (**Figure 2**) [5–7] was originally developed in Europe under the name of "ALF-X", and then sold to US company TransEnterix, Inc. It received CE mark and cleared FDA for major laparoscopic surgery. The Senhance system has three independent robotic arms for instruments and camera. Each arm stands on the floor, has long beam as seen in **Figure 2**. Various types of the forceps are available and can be attached to the robotic arms. Unique features which are different from da Vinci are gaze control system of camera and force feedback. At the control cockpit, the eye motion of the operator is monitored and is used for the camera motion. If the operator moves head forward, the camera moves closer to the object. The company claims cost effectiveness as other emerging robot company than intuitive surgical do so [7].

2.2 Versius surgical robotic system

Versius surgical robotics system (CMR Surgical Ltd., UK) also contains independent robotic arms for each instruments, but the size of the robotic arms are designed smaller (**Figure 3**). As the foot print of each robotic arm is 38 × 38 cm, it is portable, does not require large space, and setting up is easy. Comparing with 8 mm da Vinci instrument, CMR provides thinner, 5.8 mm instrument with wrist. It is under development, and not yet CE Marked nor 510(k) cleared.

2.3 Verb surgical

Johnson & Johnson (Ethicon) and Google (Verily Life Sciences) have jointly established Verb Surgical Inc. (US). Their goal is not only robotics but also

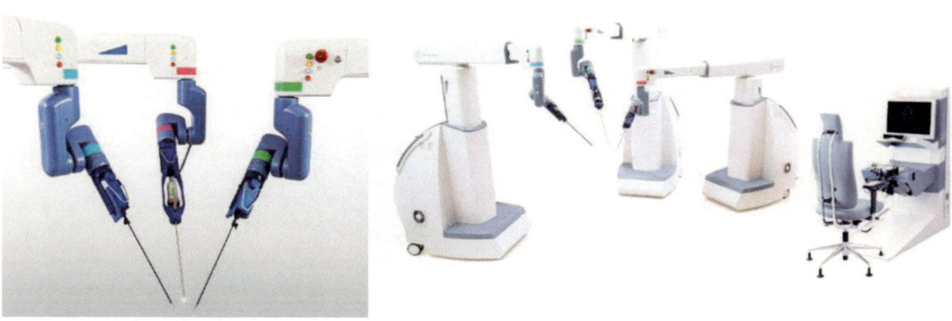

Figure 2.
Senhance surgical robotic system (©2018 TransEnterix, Inc.).

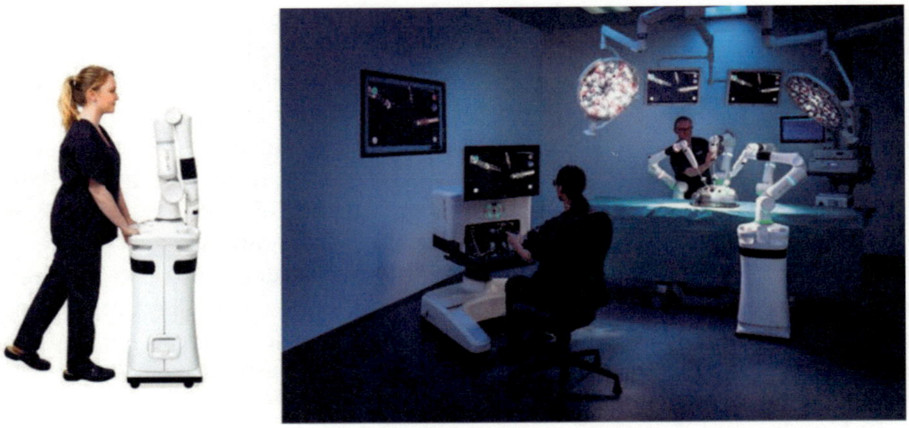

Figure 3.
Versius surgical robotic system (©2018 CMR Surgical Ltd., UK).

visualization, advanced instrumentation, data analytics, and connectivity. The details of the appearance of the robot, function, cost, etc. have not been published.

2.4 MiroSurge system

German aerospace center (DLR) developed MiroSurge system (**Figure 4**) [8, 9]. It also has independent, light weight, and compact robotic arms for each instrument, which could be fixed directly on the operating bed. Force feedback feature is implemented to the instruments. Unique feature is that the operator can move the robotic arm directly by hand touching the arm. By using this function, for example, an assistant operator can easily make a room at bed side. Medtronic is licensed this robot.

2.5 da Vinci SP

da Vinci SP (Intuitive Surgical) is a single port surgical system [10–13]. A camera and three 6-mm instruments are bundled inside a 25-mm cannula. Thus, they can be inserted into the patient body from single incision. Each instrument has seven degrees of freedom, including "elbow" and "shoulder". The camera also has multi-bending neck, so that the camera head movement is independent of instruments, and operator can look down the devices. Although initial position of

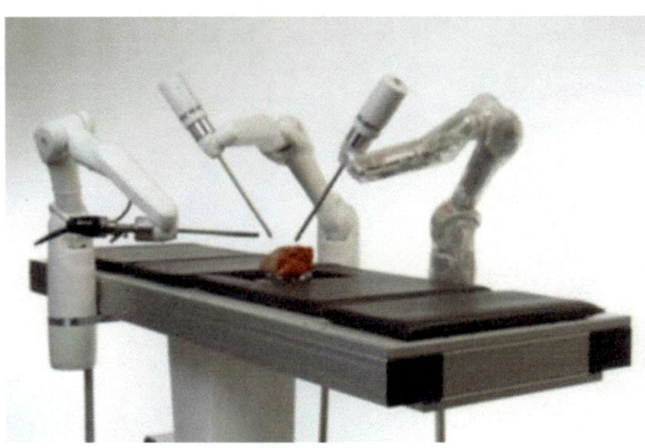

Figure 4.
MiroSurge system. Reprinted by permission from Springer Nature: Springer Nature [8].

the instruments inside the cannula is straight, the "elbow" and "shoulder" make triangulation possible inside the body. It has cleared FDA for urologic procedures. The other applications which the company is aiming at are rectum [11], laryngeal [12, 13] (through natural orifice), and other abdominal procedures.

2.6 SPORT surgical system

SPORT surgical system (TITAN Medical, Canada) is also a single port surgical system. It has two articulating instruments and a camera, in a cannula (**Figure 5**). It is under development, and the company expects its FDA clearance in 2019.

2.7 Endoscope holding robot

In the history of the surgical robot, AESOP (Computer Motion, Inc., US) [15], an endoscope holding robot, was one of the pioneers, which was launched in 1994. Although AESOP discontinued, there are some new camera holding robots. Their purpose is mainly to solve the issue of human resources in hospital. Viky (EndoControl, France) [16] is a compact camera holder which can be mounted on the operation bed (**Figure 6**). Freehand (Freehand 2010 Ltd., UK) [17] is also mounted on bed. SoloAssist (AKTORmed, Germany) [18], MTG-H100 (Hiwin Technologies Corp, Taiwan), and EMARO (Riverfield Inc., Japan) stands on the floor. Various control methods are employed, such as voice, head movement, and joystick.

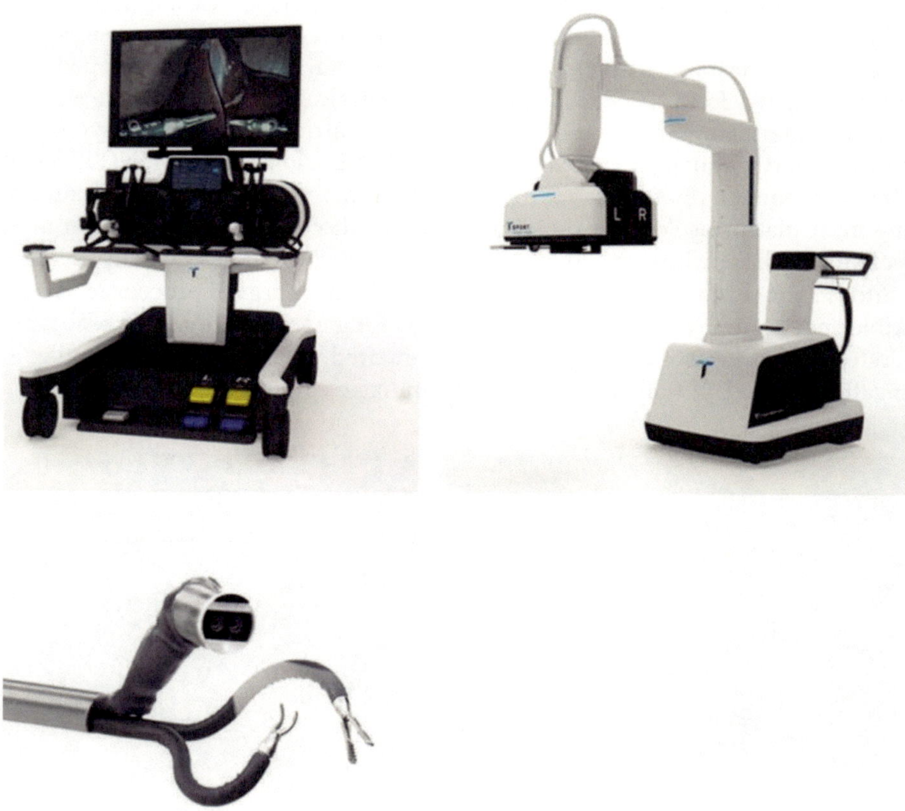

Figure 5.
SPORT surgical system. Reprinted by permission from Springer Nature: Springer Nature [14].

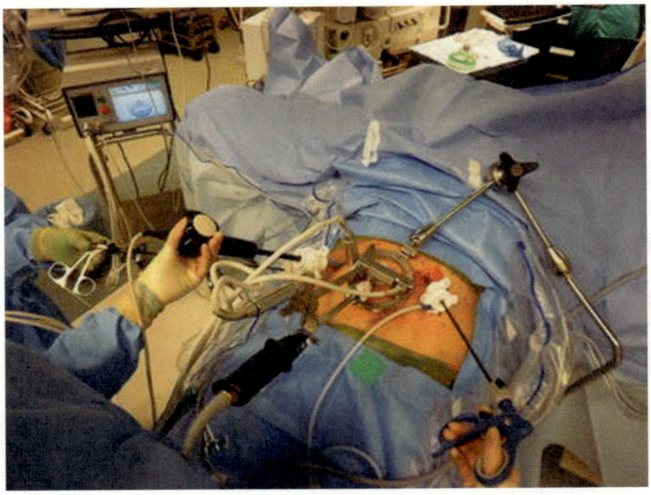

Figure 6.
Viky, reprinted by permission from Springer Nature: Springer Nature [16].

3. Robotics for the flexible endoscopic surgery

Natural orifice transluminal endoscopic surgery (NOTES) was introduced in 2004 [19]. It is the surgery using flexible endoscope instead of rigid laparoscope. As access to the lesion is through the natural orifice (mouth and anus), no incision on the patient skin, but on the organ inside body such as gastrointestinal wall instead is required. Conventional flexible endoscopes and instruments were not enough effective to perform this surgical procedure. So, several companies developed multi-tasking platform [20–25] (**Figure 7**). They basically contain flexible endoscope, articulating instruments, and grasping and cutting devices. They were not motorized, but manually actuated using wire transmission. However, NOTES is still in the experimental phase because this procedure was still technically difficult even using those platforms. Most of those platforms are discontinued. However, if new, effective device were introduced in the future, NOTES could be clinically accepted.

Endoscopic submucosal dissection (ESD) is another surgical procedure using flexible endoscope [28, 29]. ESD is applied only for gastrointestinal mucosal cancer. Therefore, it has limited coverage of organ compared with NOTES. ESD has been clinically accepted and prevailing especially in Asian countries. Although ESD

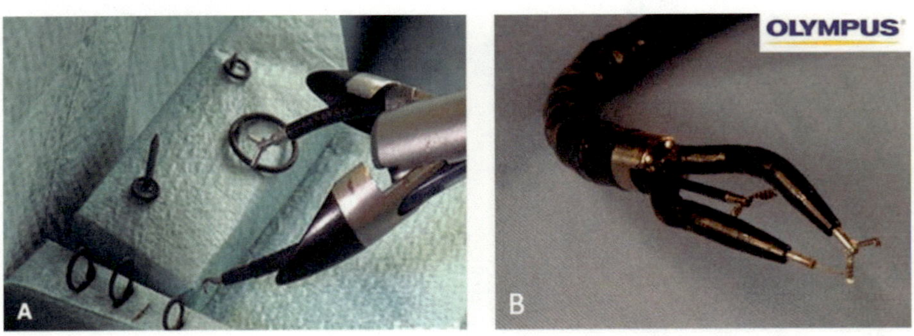

Figure 7.
Examples of manually driven multi-tasking platform. (A) ANUBISCOPE (IRCAD & Karl Storz Endoskope), reprinted by permission from Springer Nature: Springer Nature [26]. (B) EndoSAMURAI (Olympus, Japan), reprinted by permission from Springer Nature: Springer Nature [27].

procedure is easier than NOTES, it still requires high skill of flexible endoscope and long training time like laparoscopy [30, 31]. Some of the recent robotic surgical systems for flexible endoscope are aiming at ESD procedure.

In this section, recent surgical robots for flexible endoscope are introduced. At present, there is no major robot in this field. But many are under development or just have been launched. We believe flexible endoscope surgery will be next major target of surgical robot industry.

3.1 STRAS

ANUBISCOPE (IRCAD & Karl Storz Endoskope) [20, 21] was developed for NOTES and ESD procedure. The system composed of a custom made flexible endoscope with two articulating instruments. It was not motor driven but manually driven system. Strasburg University jointly developed motorized version, STRAS with Karl Storz and IRCAD [32–35]. By using vision computation technology, they applied automated target tracking [32] and position detection of the instruments [33]. This project is still in the phase of academic research. Some animal trials have been carried out [34, 35].

3.2 Endomaster

Endomaster (Endomaster Pte Ltd., Singapore) has also two articulating robotic instruments. It has "shoulder" and "elbow" joints in its instruments instead that all other platforms have consecutive bending section. The prototype (**Figure 8**) uses a conventional two channel endoscope but latest version uses custom made

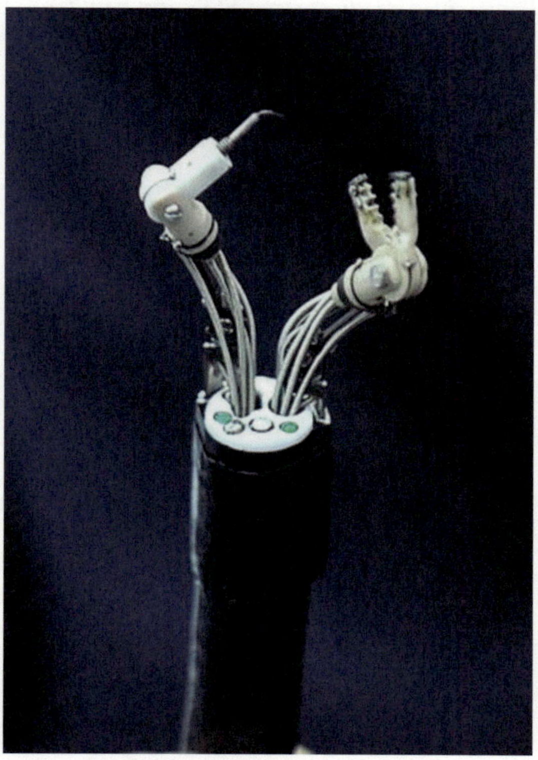

Figure 8.
EndoMaster prototype, reprinted by permission from Springer Nature: Springer Nature [36].

endoscope. This company is a spin-off of Nanyang Technological University, Singapore. HOYA Corporation, Japan, one of the endoscope manufacturers joined the project. It is still under development. ESD, endoscopic full thickness dissection, NOTES trials in animal model, and a human trial have been carried out [36–40].

3.3 Medrobotics

Flex robotic system (Medrobotics Corporation, US) has also two 4-mm articulating arm and endoscope (**Figure 9**). Unique feature is the snake-like endoscope [41–44]. By using two sets of shape-locking sheath, the endoscope can move follow-the-leader manner like snake. As the length of the endoscope is short, it can be applied for larynx, rectum from natural orifice, and percutaneously abdominal cavity. Flex robotic system has already cleared FDA for colorectal surgery.

3.4 K-Flex

Korea Advanced Institute of Science and Technology (KAIST), South Korea has been developing K-Flex [45]. Two 3.7-mm articulating instruments and an endoscope are in a flexible sheath. The sheath has wire driven bending section at the end. This bending section has two independently controllable bending parts, so that view angle can be changed. They established a spin-off company, EasyEndo Surgical Inc., to commercialize this system.

3.5 Monarch platform

Auris Health, Inc. (US) is a potential company which can develop flexible endoscopic robot [46]. They have already cleared FDA and launched the Monarch platform in 2018, which is a bronchoscopy treatment robot. They previously acquired Hansen Medical, which had technology for bending catheter for cardiovascular use. At the moment, they focus on lung treatment.

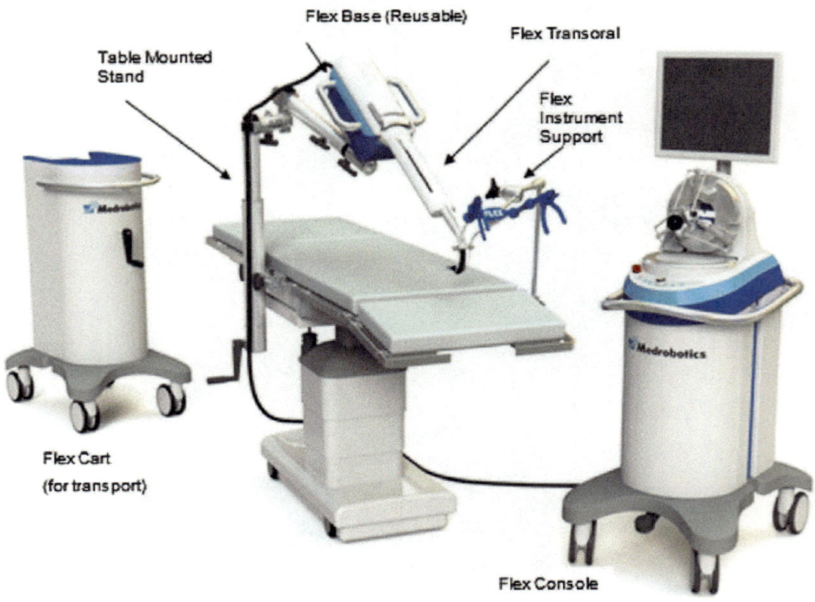

Figure 9.
Flex robotic system, reprinted by permission from Springer Nature: Springer Nature [41].

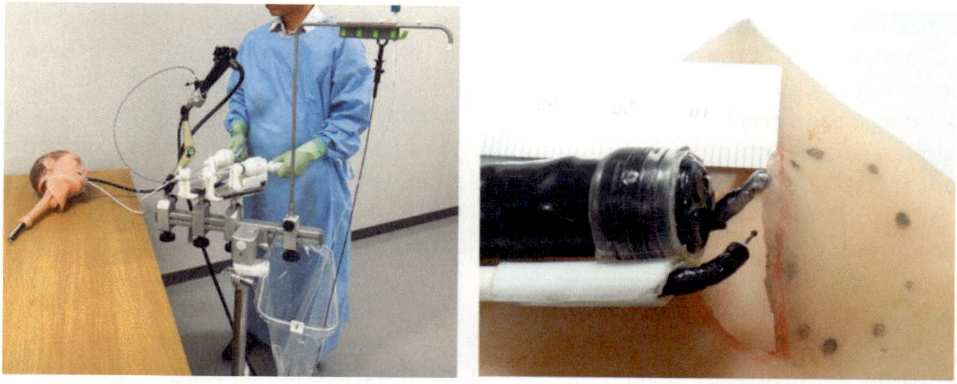

Figure 10.
ESD platform (manually driven) of Kyushu University, Japan.

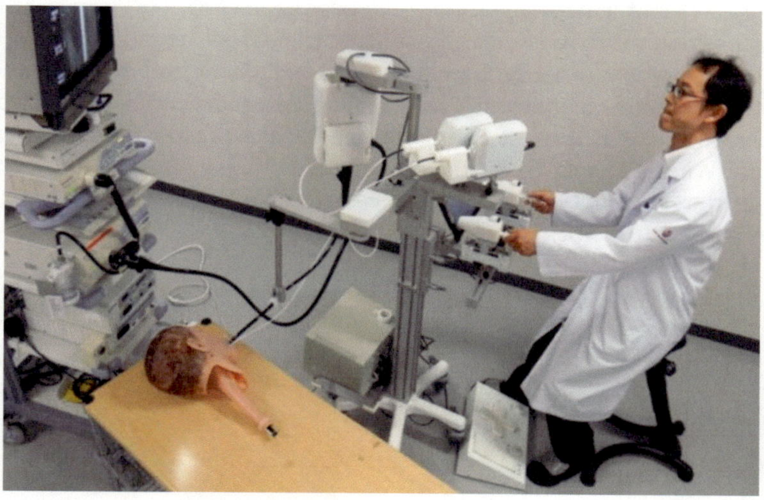

Figure 11.
ESD platform (motorized) of Kyushu University, Japan.

3.6 Kyushu University ESD robot

We have also been developing flexible endoscopic platforms for ESD in manually driven version [47, 48] (**Figure 10**) and motorized version [49] (**Figure 11**). They composed of conventional flexible endoscope, two 2.6-mm articulating instruments, and an additional channel. By using standard endoscope for ESD, total system cost is minimized. The diameter of instruments is very thin because the standard endoscope has 2.8 mm channel. Control part on a stand is designed, so that both handles of the instruments and endoscope are close to the operator. Animal experiments have been carried out [47, 48].

4. Other robotic application

4.1 Teleoperation

Telesurgery is one of the possible applications of surgical robot for the purpose of medicine in rural area, space, and battle field. In principle of surgical robot, master controller (operator site) and surgical robot (patient site) are connected only by signal. So even if the whole system is in a room like da Vinci, they are teleoperation robot in nature. In the case of long distance between operator site and patient site, delay in the signal transmission is not negligible. Therefore, fast transmission lines are chosen and employed. Marescaux et al. demonstrated telesurgery experiment on human patient between US and France [50]. We also have also successfully carried out animal telesurgery experiments several times between Japan and Korea, Japan and Thailand by using our own robot system (**Figure 12**) [51, 52]. In this study, we have employed relatively low cost ISDN line and low latency CODEC technology.

4.2 MRI compatible robot

Anatomy identification is sometimes difficult during laparoscopic surgery. If surgeon can see vessel, nerve, and lesion under the organ surface, it will be strong merit for safety and quality of the operation. For this purpose, we used intraoperative open bore type MRI for real-time image acquisition and developed a laparoscopic surgical robot which can be placed inside the MRI gantry (**Figure 13**) [53]. As MRI has strong magnetic field, no magnetic metal such as stainless steel cannot be used. Our robot was made of mainly engineering plastic and titanium alloy. Also, we chose ultrasonic motors instead of magnetic motors. The system consists of two forceps and a camera. Additionally, needle insertion device can be attached. The surgeon console display shows the camera view, pre-operative MR image, and intraoperative real-time MR image. We have successfully demonstrated animal experiment by live porcine model.

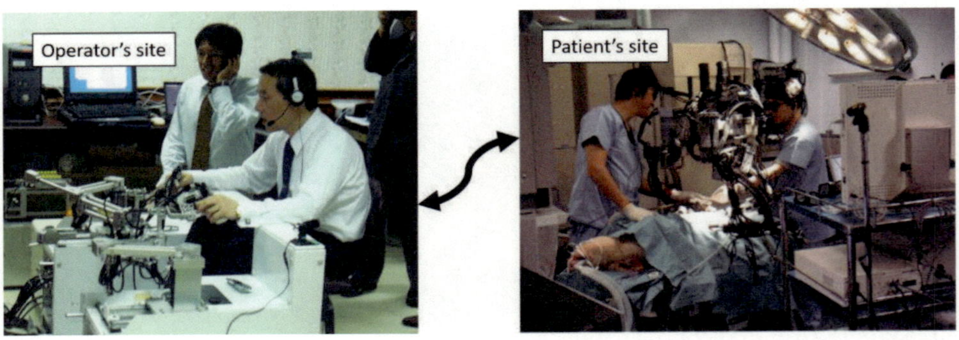

Figure 12.
(Left) Master console (right) patient site of the teleoperation robot.

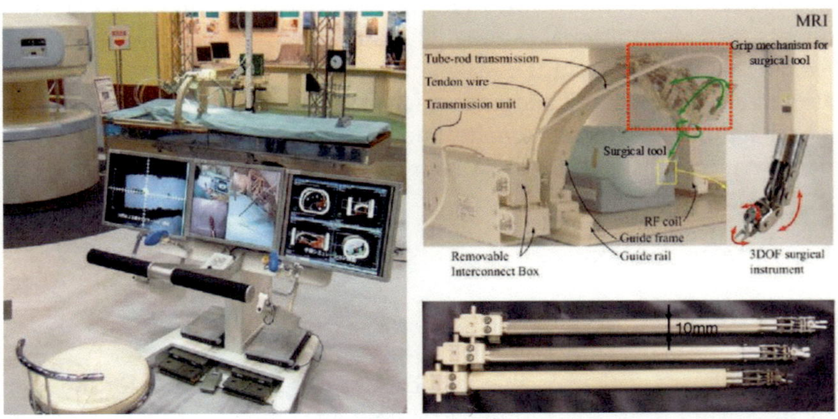

Figure 13.
MRI image-guided surgical system, reprinted by permission from Springer Nature: Springer Nature [53].

5. Navigation

Navigation in surgery includes various techniques. In brain and ENT surgery where the organ deformation are relatively small, the navigation system which detects the real-time position of the instrument in the preoperative three-dimensional image by using optical position sensors is often used. In laparoscopic surgery, as the organ movement is large, such precise position detection is not required. But sometimes surgeon requires to refer to the segmented preoperative image during the procedure in order to confirm anatomical structure. The problem was that it is very difficult to compare current two-dimensional camera image and preoperative three-dimensional image. In order to solve this problem, we have developed real-time viewer software and sensor system especially for da Vinci partial nephrectomy (**Figure 14**) [54, 55]. This system detects the robot camera angle by position sensor mounted to the da Vinci arm by our own attachment (because da Vinci does not allow to output such data). According to the camera angle, the system computes corresponding view in the three-dimensional preoperative image and displays at the small sub-display under the main display. By this navigation system, the surgeon can see the preoperative image in the same angle of current camera image. We found it very useful, and it is clinically used every time in our hospital.

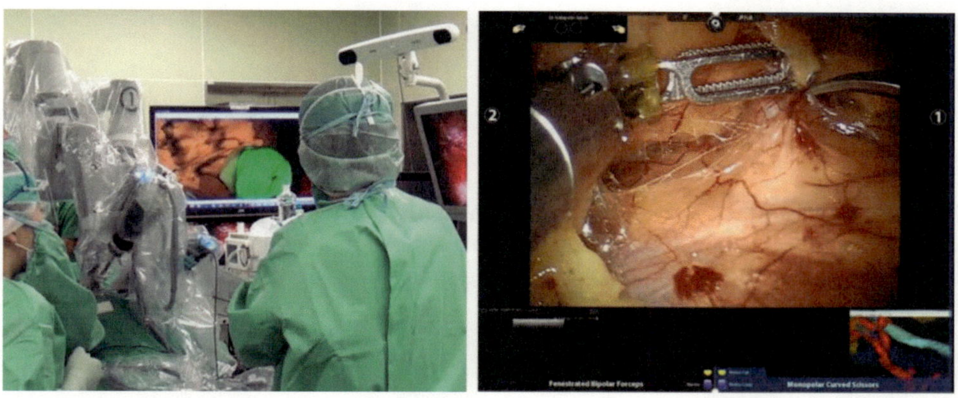

Figure 14.
Navigation system for da Vinci surgery.

6. Training

Training in laparoscopic surgery is important for surgeons. Also, studies about effective training method are important for better learning curve. There are many surgical simulators using computer graphics, rubber phantom, and harvested animal organ. However, measuring surgical skill quantitatively was very difficult. Quantification of skill is important not only for qualifying each surgeon but also for evaluating the effectiveness of training method. We have developed a suture simulator and evaluation software (**Figure 15**) [56, 57]. The phantom mimicking small intestine, made of four layers and string braided rubber, is used for the task. The task is anastomosis of the defect on the intestine by three interrupted sutures. The result is evaluated by five category including completion time, air leakage test, etc. The trainees can be fed back each time by score. Scoring system was developed using data previously obtained from skilled surgeons performing suture on this phantom. By using this simulator, significant difference between the trainees' scores before and after training was observed [57].

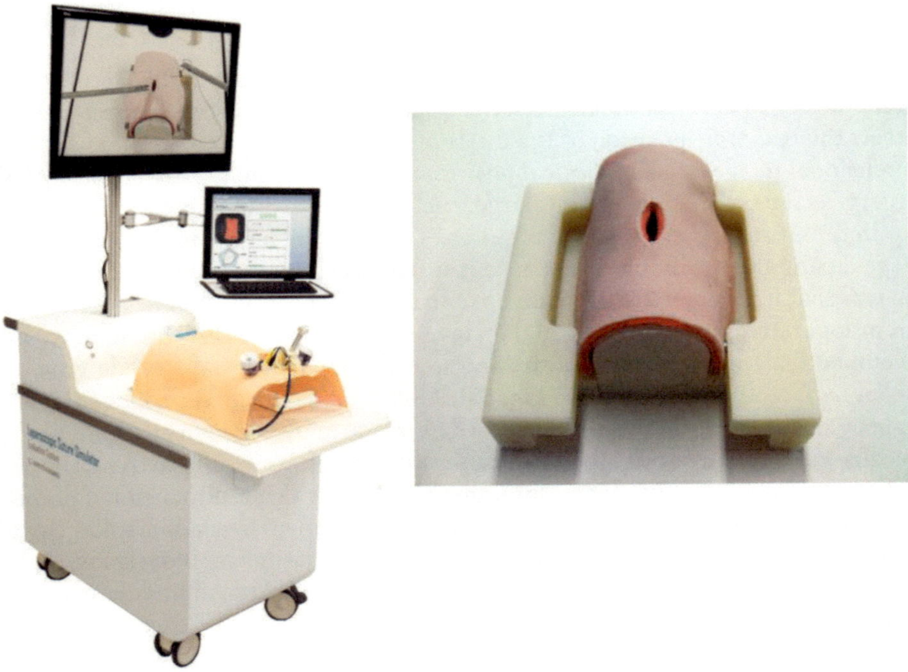

Figure 15.
Training simulator.

7. Conclusion

In this chapter, we introduced current and near future available laparoscopic/flexible endoscopic surgical robots, examples of other advanced robotic applications, and technology of navigation and training.

Conflict of interest

Ryu Nakadate and Makoto Hashizume received researching fund from Hogy Medical Co Ltd., Japan. This work was partially supported by JSPS KAKENHI Grant Number 16H03195.

DOI: http://dx.doi.org/10.5772/intechopen.82191

Author details

Ryu Nakadate[1] and Makoto Hashizume[2]*

1 Center for Advanced Medical Innovation, Kyushu University, Fukuoka, Japan

2 Kitakyushu Chuo Hospital, Fukuoka, Japan

*Address all correspondence to: mhashi@dem.med.kyushu-u.ac.jp

References

[1] Jourdan IC, Dutson E, Garcia A, Vleugels T, Leroy J, Mutter D, et al. Stereoscopic vision provides a significant advantage for precision robotic laparoscopy. British Journal of Surgery. 2004;**91**:879-885. DOI: 10.1002/bjs.4549

[2] Gallagher AG, McClure N, McGuigan J, Ritchie K, Sheehy NP. An ergonomic analysis of the fulcrum effect in the acquisition of endoscopic skills. Endoscopy. 1998;**30**:617-620. DOI: 10.1055/s-2007-1001366

[3] Guthart GS, Salisbury JK. The Intuitive/sup TM/telesurgery system: Overview and application. In: Proceedings of the IEEE International Conference on Robotics and Automation (ICRA2000); San Francisco. 2000. pp. 618-621. DOI: 10.1109/ROBOT.2000.844121

[4] Intuitive Surgical, Inc., Investor Presentation August 2018 [Internet]. 2018. Available from: https://isrg.intuitive.com/static-files/8bbddc9e-579c-47a1-ac91-fabe26e5e278 [Accessed: 14-09-2018]

[5] Gueli Alletti S, Perrone E, Cianci S, Rossitto C, Monterossi G, Bernardini F, et al. 3 mm Senhance robotic hysterectomy: A step towards future perspectives. Journal of Robotic Surgery. 2018;**12**:575-577. DOI: 10.1007/s11701-018-0778-5

[6] Hutchins AR, Manson RJ, Lerebours R, Farjat AE, Cox ML, Mann BP, et al. Objective assessment of the early stages of the learning curve for the senhance surgical robotic system. Journal of Surgical Education. 2018. DOI: 10.1016/j.jsurg.2018.06.026

[7] Rossitto C, Alletti SG, Romano F, Fiore A, Coretti S, Oradei M, et al. Use of robot-specific resources and operating room times: The case of Telelap Alf-X robotic hysterectomy. The International Journal of Medical Robotics and Computer Assisted Surgery. 2016;**12**:613-619. DOI: 10.1002/rcs.1724

[8] Hagn U, Konietschke R, Tobergte A, Nickl M, Jörg S, Kübler B, et al. DLR MiroSurge: A versatile system for research in endoscopic telesurgery. International Journal of Computer Assisted Radiology and Surgery. 2010;**5**:183-193. DOI: 10.1007/s11548-009-0372-4

[9] Konietschke R, Hagn U, Nickl M, Jorg S, Tobergte A, Passig G, et al. The DLR MiroSurge—A robotic system for surgery. In: Proceedings of the IEEE International Conference on Robotics and Automation (ICRA2009); Kobe. 2009. pp. 1589-1590. DOI: 10.1109/ROBOT.2009.5152361

[10] Ramirez D, Maurice MJ, Kaouk JH. Robotic single-port surgery: Paving the way for the future. Urology. 2016;**95**:5-10. DOI: 10.1016/j.urology.2016.05.013

[11] Marks J, Ng S, Mak T. Robotic transanal surgery (RTAS) with utilization of a next-generation single-port system: A cadaveric feasibility study. Techniques in Coloproctology. 2017;**21**:541-545. DOI: 10.1007/s10151-017-1655-3

[12] Tateya I, Koh YW, Tsang RK, Hong SS, Uozumi R, Kishimoto Y, et al. Flexible next-generation robotic surgical system for transoral endoscopic hypopharyngectomy: A comparative preclinical study. Head & Neck. 2018;**40**:16-23. DOI: 10.1002/hed.24868

[13] Chen MM, Orosco RK, Lim GC, Holsinger FC. Improved transoral dissection of the tongue base with a next-generation robotic surgical system. The Laryngoscope. 2018;**128**:78-83. DOI: 10.1002/lary.26649

[14] Peters BS, Armijo PR, Krause C, et al. Review of emerging surgical robotic technology. Surgical Endoscopy. 2018;**32**:1636-1655. DOI: 10.1007/s00464-018-6079-2

[15] Mettler L, Ibrahim M, Jonat W. One year of experience working with the aid of a robotic assistant (the voice-controlled optic holder AESOP) in gynaecological endoscopic surgery. Human Reproduction. 1998;**13**: 2748-2750. DOI: 10.1093/humrep/13.10.2748

[16] Gumbs AA, Croner R, Rodriguez A, Zuker N, Perrakis A, Gayet B. 200 Consecutive laparoscopic pancreatic resections performed with a robotically controlled laparoscope holder. Surgical Endoscopy. 2013;**27**:3781-3791. DOI: 10.1007/s00464-013-2969-5

[17] Stolzenburg J-U, Franz T, Kallidonis P, Minh D, Dietel A, Hicks J, et al. Comparison of the FreeHand® robotic camera holder with human assistants during endoscopic extraperitoneal radical prostatectomy. BJU International. 2011;**107**:970-974. DOI: 10.1111/j.1464-410X.2010.09656.x

[18] Ohmura Y, Nakagawa M, Suzuki H, Kotani K, Teramoto A. Feasibility and usefulness of a joystick-guided robotic scope holder (soloassist) in laparoscopic surgery. Visceral Medicine. 2018;**34**:37-44. DOI: 10.1159/000485524

[19] Kalloo AN, Singh VK, Jagannath SB, Niiyama H, Hill SL, Vaughn CA, et al. Flexible transgastric peritoneoscopy: A novel approach to diagnostic and therapeutic interventions in the peritoneal cavity. Gastrointestinal Endoscopy. 2004;**60**:114-117

[20] Dallemagne B, Marescaux J. The ANUBISTM project. Minimally Invasive Therapy & Allied Technologies. 2010;**19**:257-261. DOI: 10.3109/13645706.2010.514741

[21] Perretta S, Dallemagne B, Barry B, Marescaux J. The ANUBISCOPE® flexible platform ready for prime time: Description of the first clinical case. Surgical Endoscopy. 2013;**27**:2630-2630. DOI: 10.1007/s00464-013-2818-6

[22] Spaun GO, Zheng B, Martinec DV, Cassera MA, Dunst CM, Swanström LL. Bimanual coordination in natural orifice transluminal endoscopic surgery: Comparing the conventional dual-channel endoscope, the R-Scope, and a novel direct-drive system. Gastrointestinal Endoscopy. 2009;**69**:e39-e45. DOI: 10.1016/j.gie.2008.12.239

[23] Thompson CC, Ryou M, Soper NJ, Hungess ES, Rothstein RI, Swanstrom LL. Evaluation of a manually driven, multitasking platform for complex endoluminal and natural orifice transluminal endoscopic surgery applications (with video). Gastrointestinal Endoscopy. 2009;**70**:121-125. DOI: 10.1016/j.gie.2008.11.007

[24] Spaun GO, Zheng B, Swanström LL. A multitasking platform for natural orifice translumenal endoscopic surgery (NOTES): A benchtop comparison of a new device for flexible endoscopic surgery and a standard dual-channel endoscope. Surgical Endoscopy. 2009;**23**:2720. DOI: 10.1007/s00464-009-0476-5

[25] Ikeda K, Sumiyama K, Tajiri H, Yasuda K, Kitano S. Evaluation of a new multitasking platform for endoscopic full-thickness resection. Gastrointestinal Endoscopy. 2011;**73**:117-122. DOI: 10.1016/j.gie.2010.09.016

[26] Diana M, Chung H, Liu KH, et al. Endoluminal surgical triangulation: Overcoming challenges of colonic endoscopic submucosal dissections using a novel flexible endoscopic surgical platform: Feasibility study in

a porcine model. Surgical Endoscopy. 2013;**27**:4130-4135. DOI: 10.1007/s00464-013-3049-6

[27] Fuchs KH, Breithaupt W. Transgastric small bowel resection with the new multitasking platform EndoSAMURAI™ for natural orifice transluminal endoscopic surgery. Surgical Endoscopy. 2012;**26**:2281-2287. DOI: 10.1007/s00464-012-2173-z

[28] Gotoda T, Kondo H, Ono H, Saito Y, Yamaguchi H, Saito D, et al. A new endoscopic mucosal resection procedure using an insulation-tipped electrosurgical knife for rectal flat lesions: Report of two cases. Gastrointestinal Endoscopy. 1999;**50**:560-563. DOI: 10.1016/S0016-5107(99)70084-2

[29] Yahagi N, Fujishiro M, Kakushima N, Kobayashi K, Hashimoto T, Oka M, et al. Endoscopic submucosal dissection for early gastric cancer using the tip of an electrosurgical snare (thin type). Digestive Endoscopy. 2004;**16**:34-38. DOI: 10.1111/j.1443-1661.2004.00313.x

[30] Deprez PH, Bergman JJ, Meisner S, Ponchon T, Repici A, Dinis-Ribeiro M, et al. Current practice with endoscopic submucosal dissection in Europe: Position statement from a panel of experts. Endoscopy. 2010;**42**:853-858. DOI: 10.1055/s-0030-1255563

[31] Fukami N. What we want for ESD is a second hand! Traction method. Gastrointestinal Endoscopy. 2013;**78**:274-276. DOI: 10.1016/j.gie.2013.04.192

[32] Ott L, Nageotte F, Zanne P, de Mathelin M. Robotic assistance to flexible endoscopy by physiological-motion tracking. IEEE Transactions on Robotics. 2011;**27**:346-359. DOI: 10.1109/TRO.2010.2098623

[33] Cabras P, Goyard D, Nageotte F, Zanne P, Doignon C. Comparison of methods for estimating the position of actuated instruments in flexible endoscopic surgery. In: Proceedings of the IEEE/RSJ International Conference on Intelligent Robots and Systems (IROS2014); Chicago. 2014. pp. 3522-3528. DOI: 10.1109/IROS.2014.6943054

[34] Zorn L, Nageotte F, Zanne P, Legner A, Dallemagne B, Marescaux J, et al. A novel telemanipulated robotic assistant for surgical endoscopy: Preclinical application to ESD. IEEE Transactions on Biomedical Engineering. 2018;**65**:797-808. DOI: 10.1109/TBME.2017.2720739

[35] Légner A, Diana M, Halvax P, Liu Y-Y, Zorn L, Zanne P, et al. Endoluminal surgical triangulation 2.0: A new flexible surgical robot. Preliminary pre-clinical results with colonic submucosal dissection. The International Journal of Medical Robotics and Computer Assisted Surgery. 2017;**13**:e1819. DOI: 10.1002/rcs.1819

[36] Chiu PWY, Phee SJ, Wang Z, Sun Z, Poon CC, Yamamoto T, et al. Feasibility of full-thickness gastric resection using master and slave transluminal endoscopic robot and closure by overstitch: A preclinical study. Surgical Endoscopy. 2014;**28**:319-324. DOI: 10.1007/s00464-013-3149-3

[37] Phee LS, Ho KY, Shabbir A, Low SC, Huynh VA, Kencana AP, et al. Endoscopic submucosal dissection of gastric lesions using a through-the-scope intuitively controlled robotics-enhanced manipulator system. Gastrointestinal Endoscopy. 2009;**69**:AB163. DOI: 10.1016/j.gie.2009.03.291

[38] Phee SJ, Ho KY, Lomanto D, Low SC, Huynh VA, Kencana AP, et al. Natural orifice transgastric

endoscopic wedge hepatic resection in an experimental model using an intuitively controlled master and slave transluminal endoscopic robot (MASTER). Surgical Endoscopy. 2010;**24**:2293-2298. DOI: 10.1007/s00464-010-0955-8

[39] Phee SJ, Reddy N, Chiu PWY, Rebala P, Rao GV, Wang Z, et al. Robot-assisted endoscopic submucosal dissection is effective in treating patients with early-stage gastric neoplasia. Clinical Gastroenterology and Hepatology. 2012;**10**:1117-1121. DOI: 10.1016/j.cgh.2012.05.019

[40] Tay G, Tan H-K, Nguyen TK, Phee SJ, Iyer NG. Use of the EndoMaster robot-assisted surgical system in transoral robotic surgery: A cadaveric study. The International Journal of Medical Robotics and Computer Assisted Surgery. 2018;**14**:e1930. DOI: 10.1002/rcs.1930

[41] Remacle M, M. N. Prasad V, Lawson G, Plisson L, Bachy V, Van der Vorst S. Transoral robotic surgery (TORS) with the medrobotics FlexTM system: First surgical application on humans. European Archives of Oto-Rhino-Laryngology. 2015;**272**:1451-1455. DOI: 10.1007/s00405-015-3532-x

[42] Funk E, Goldenberg D, Goyal N. Demonstration of transoral robotic supraglottic laryngectomy and total laryngectomy in cadaveric specimens using the medrobotics flex system. Head & Neck. 2017;**39**:1218-1225. DOI: 10.1002/hed.24746

[43] Atallah S, Hodges A, Larach SW. Direct target NOTES: Prospective applications for next generation robotic platforms. Techniques in Coloproctology. 2018;**22**:363-371. DOI: 10.1007/s10151-018-1788-z

[44] Rivera-Serrano CM, Johnson P, Zubiate B, Kuenzler R, Choset H, Zenati M, et al. A transoral highly flexible robot. The Laryngoscope. 2012;**122**:1067-1071. DOI: 10.1002/lary.23237

[45] Hwang M, Kwon D-S. Strong continuum manipulator for flexible endoscopic surgery. In: Proceedings of 10th Hamlyn Symposium on Medical Robotics (HSMR2017); London. 2017. pp. 63-64

[46] Auris Health. Inc. [Internet]. 2018. Available from: https://www.aurishealth.com/home [Accessed: 14-09-2018]

[47] Nakadate R, Nakamura S, Moriyama T, Kenmotsu H, Oguri S, Arata J, et al. Gastric endoscopic submucosal dissection using novel 2.6 mm articulating devices: An ex vivo comparative and in vivo feasibility study. Endoscopy. 2015;**47**:820-824. DOI: 10.1055/s-0034-1391438

[48] Okamoto Y, Nakadate R, Nakamura S, Arata J, Oguri S, Moriyama T, et al. Colorectal endoscopic submucosal dissection using novel articulating devices: A comparative study in a live porcine model. Surgical Endoscopy. 2018. DOI: 10.1007/s00464-018-6408-5

[49] Iwasa T, Nakadate R, Onogi S, Okamoto Y, Arata J, Oguri S, et al. A new robotic-assisted flexible endoscope with single-hand control: Endoscopic submucosal dissection in the ex vivo porcine stomach. Surgical Endoscopy. 2018;**32**:3386-3392. DOI: 10.1007/s00464-018-6188-y

[50] Marescaux J, Leroy J, Gagner M, Rubino F, Mutter D, Vix M, et al. Transatlantic robot-assisted telesurgery. Nature. 2001;**413**:379-380. DOI: 10.1038/35096636

[51] Arata J, Takahashi H, Pitakwatchara P, Warisawa S, Tanoue K, Konishi K,

et al. A remote surgery experiment between Japan and Thailand over Internet using a low latency CODEC system. In: Proceedings of the IEEE International Conference on Robotics and Automation (ICRA2007); Roma. 2007. pp. 953-959. DOI: 10.1109/ROBOT.2007.363108

[52] Arata J, Takahashi H, Yasunaka S, Onda K, Tanaka K, Sugita N, et al. Impact of network time-delay and force feedback on tele-surgery. International Journal of Computer Assisted Radiology and Surgery. 2008;**3**:371-378. DOI: 10.1007/s11548-008-0228-3

[53] Hashizume M, Yasunaga T, Tanoue K, Ieiri S, Konishi K, Kishi K, et al. New real-time MR image-guided surgical robotic system for minimally invasive precision surgery. International Journal of Computer Assisted Radiology and Surgery. 2008;**2**:317-325. DOI: 10.1007/s11548-007-0146-9

[54] Kobayashi S, Cho B, Tatsugami K, Hashizume M, Eto M. Surgical navigation using intuitive image-to-patient registration for robot-assisted partial nephrectomy: Clinical feasibility study. International Journal of Computer Assisted Radiology and Surgery. 2017;**12**:S263-S264. DOI: 10.1007/s11548-017-1588-3

[55] Kobayashi S, Cho B, Tatsugami K, Hashizume M, Eto M. Surgical navigation using intuitive image-to-patient registration for robot-assisted partial nephrectomy: Clinical feasibility study. Journal of Endourology. 2017;**31**(S2):V3-V6. DOI: 10.1089/end.2017.29029.abstracts

[56] Uemura M, Yamashita M, Tomikawa M, Obata S, Souzaki R, Ieiri S, et al. Objective assessment of the suture ligature method for the laparoscopic intestinal anastomosis model using a new computerized system. Surgical Endoscopy. 2015;**29**:444-452. DOI: 10.1007/s00464-014-3681-9

[57] Takeoka T, Takiguchi S, Uemura M, Miyazaki Y, Takahashi T, Kurokawa Y, et al. Assessment potential of a new suture simulator in laparoscopic surgical skills training. Minimally Invasive Therapy & Allied Technologies. 2017;**26**:338-345. DOI: 10.1080/13645706.2017.1312456